HEAL
YOUR DISC
END
YOUR PAIN

How Regenerative Medicine
Can Save Your Spine

HEAL
YOUR DISC
END
YOUR PAIN

GREGORY E. LUTZ, MD

Disclaimer: This book does not provide medical advice.

The content—including but not limited to text, graphics, images, and other material—contained in this book is for informational purposes only. None of the information is intended to be a substitute for personal professional medical advice, diagnosis, or treatment. Before undertaking a new healthcare regimen, always seek the advice of a physician or other qualified healthcare provider with any questions you may have regarding a medical condition or treatment; and do not disregard professional medical advice or delay seeking it because of something you have read in this book.

LIONCREST
PUBLISHING

Heal Your Disc, End Your Pain

How Regenerative Medicine Can Save Your Spine

ISBN 978-1-5445-3721-4 Hardcover

978-1-5445-3722-1 Paperback

978-1-5445-3723-8 Ebook

978-1-5445-3823-5 Audiobook

To Paula,

My love and inspiration.

CONTENTS

The Regenerative SportsCare Foundation (RSF) is a 501(c)(3) charitable organization whose mission is TO FIND A CURE FOR DEGENERATIVE DISC DISEASE.

All proceeds from the sale of this book will go to RSF to fund research to help heal your disc and end your pain.

Throughout this book, you'll learn about the research RSF and others have carried out to help patients find clinically studied, safer, and more effective treatments to relieve their back pain and restore spinal health.

By purchasing a copy of this book, you are helping to fund critical research in the promising field of regenerative medicine.

To learn more about the Regenerative SportsCare Foundation, including our current studies, please visit www.regensports care.com/foundation/.

A NOTE TO YOU

I've never written a book before. I always wanted to but just never had the time. Between balancing a very busy clinical practice and family responsibilities, there was no chance to stop, collect my thoughts, and write. I'm sure there are many physicians who feel that way during their careers.

In their decades of clinical experience managing patients with a specific medical condition, they learn something special that maybe no one else has yet noticed, a "nugget" of information that could potentially change the treatment paradigm for that condition and make life better for everyone. But due to their busy schedules or lack of resources, they are never able to share their discovery beyond the walls of their own practice.

That could have very well been my story, too, if not for COVID. My clinical practice was directly in the middle of the it, in the heart of New York City, and the pandemic was a terrible experience for us all. We were shut down for over three months by state mandate, because all healthcare resources had to focus on addressing the virus.

Without that pandemic pause, I don't think this book would have been written. It created the "hard stop" that finally gave me the time I needed to share with you my nugget of wisdom regarding how I believe we can better manage back pain.

While the pandemic was tragic, the shutdown gave me time to think, reminding me why I became a physician and what I find so compelling about this noble profession—caring for patients and helping them heal from their wounds.

We endure many types of "wounds" in life—psychological, emotional, and physical. The wound you'll learn about in this book is in your spine, more specifically in your disc.

I'll explain that chronic lower back pain is usually nothing more than an unhealed wound in your disc, which can be treated simply and effectively with your own cells. Not drugs, not surgery—just your own cells. That is the nugget I would like to share with you. Hopefully this knowledge will help you or a loved one find an answer to your chronic lower back pain.

—Dr. Greg

CHAPTER 1

MY PATH TOWARDS REGENERATIVE MEDICINE

"Progress is impossible without change, and those who cannot change their minds cannot change anything."

—GEORGE BERNARD SHAW

I grew up in a medical family. My father was a physician with a home office where my mother, a nurse, worked alongside him. When they were not working or traveling, they enjoyed entertaining, especially other physicians—and my mother was a marvelous cook. I spent countless evenings seated at our dining room table, listening to them "talk shop" over leisurely dinners. My father was passionate about patient care. On Sundays, while we watched football games, my dad would lie prone on the living room carpet, surrounded by stacks of medical journals he was reading and index cards filled with handwritten notes. When I was in college, he and I cowrote a paper on abnormal brain-wave patterns in patients with agoraphobia, an anxiety disorder. Those experiences instilled in me great respect and admiration for the field of medicine; it was clear to me that medicine is a calling, and I wanted to be a part of that world of care and healing. As a matter of fact, I was not the only one to heed the call. All of my siblings are physicians, and now members of the next generation of our family are on their way into medicine as well.

When I was accepted into medical school, my parents and I were over the moon. I had my heart set on becoming an orthopedic surgeon. The first two years focused primarily on book learning and testing. The third and fourth years were spent in practical electives, rotating through a variety of specialties ("rotations") where we actually interacted with and treated patients under supervision. As you might imagine, by the fourth year, I couldn't wait to finally begin my orthopedic rotation.

It was 1987, Ronald Reagan was president, the New York Giants had won the Super Bowl, and I was in my final year of medical school. Beth was my very first orthopedic patient.

It was a challenge even to examine her; not only was she in a great deal of pain, but she was also upset and exhausted. Beth was relatively young—in her forties—a wife and mom of four kids, who had suffered for years from chronic lower back pain (CLBP) due to degenerative disc disease (DDD). She had tried all the traditional treatments: oral medication, physical therapy, chiropractic care, spinal injections, and time—none of which had given her any sustained relief. Frustrated, she went to a spine surgeon who told her he could "fix" her problem by fusing her spine with screws and rods.

Following the spinal fusion, Beth was in even worse pain than before. Implants in the spine can sometimes become a breeding ground for bacterial growth. The screws that held Beth's spine together had become infected, and the only way to eradicate the infection was for her to undergo a second spinal surgery to remove the spinal implants and irrigate the wound with antibiotics. I walked into Beth's room just after that second surgery.

Beth saw me—a medical student—as a nuisance, the source of yet another exam requiring her to gingerly shift positions. Her distress was understandable. After all, she was recovering from her second spinal surgery in less than two weeks, and she was required to take daily pain medication, which worsened her depression. She would now need to spend several more weeks bedridden, receiving massive doses of intravenous antibiotics to try and fight the infection. Even if her recovery progressed as planned and hoped, she would still need to undergo a third spinal surgery to redo the fusion and stabilize her spine so that she could walk again.

In the 1980s, the use of spinal implants usually involved hooks and rods and was typically reserved for patients who had scoliosis, a curvature of the spine. A spine bone screw and plate system was not the typical surgery for patients with lower back pain from degenerative discs. At that time, there was a lot of experimentation going on with these types of spinal implants.[1] New pedicle screw systems and surgical techniques were being invented and reinvented with the goal of achieving a solid spinal fusion. Practitioners hoped the elimination of motion and load on degenerative discs would relieve patients' back pain.

Dr. Art Steffee, who is considered by many to be the father of modern spine surgery, invented a pedicle screw system in 1982 that could be used in the lower back. This spine stabilizing system is what Beth had received. In his initial publication, Dr. Steffee mentioned a 90 percent "success rate." However, he subsequently admitted that his follow-up period was too short.

Out of 120 patients, there were seven deep infections, two nerve injuries, eight broken screws, and five loose screws that had to be removed. So if you add up these complications, his reported 90 percent success rate was optimistic at best. Even so, he later founded a spine implant company called Acromed and sold it to DePuy in 1998 for $325 million.

Beth was one of the early pedicle screw fusion cases. She had exhausted all of the traditional conservative treatments at that time without success and, like many patients in her circumstance, she had to make a very difficult decision: should she continue to live with unbearable pain, or should she take the risk of undergoing a relatively new type of spinal fusion surgery?

The day I met Beth, I performed the best exam that I could under the circumstances. As I walked home that evening, I couldn't stop thinking about her and her suffering. Here was a woman who, just like my own mom, was responsible for raising four children. Her pain was interfering with her family life, and she'd undergone surgery in the hope of reclaiming her mobility. Now, she was fighting for her life.

The next morning, I performed my rounds. When I reached Beth's room, her bed was empty. Curious, I went to the nurse's station to ask what room they'd moved her to. "Beth died last night," the nurse responded apologetically. The pen I was holding fell from my hand; those were not the words I'd expected to hear. I felt shocked and nauseous.

Overnight, Beth had developed a blood clot that had traveled to her lungs, killing her instantly—this is called a pulmonary embolism. This complication was a direct result of her two recent surgeries, the infection she was fighting, and the bed-rest her recovery required. She probably had not needed such an aggressive spinal surgery, but she'd decided to proceed, and now she was dead. It was the worst outcome possible.

I knew there had to have been a safer way to treat chronic lower back pain patients like Beth. I did not yet know what that solution would be, but even as a green medical student, I sensed that fusions could not be the answer for most patients suffering from CLBP. There had to be something better than cutting a disc out and fusing the spine with screws and rods.

Looking back, I can see now how the medical establishment failed Beth twice: first, when she tried conservative treatments that were ineffectual; and second, when she underwent a spinal fusion because there was nothing better to offer her. I carried my experience with Beth throughout my entire professional career, and it proved to be pivotal in pursuing a path outside of orthopedic surgery.

While outcomes like Beth's are thankfully rare, that experience motivated me to devote a large portion of my career to preventing other patients from suffering the same fate. It led me to a lesser-known medical specialty and answers in the unlikeliest of places. Most importantly, it caused me to find a *safe* potential solution for the type of chronic, disabling back pain that had ultimately led to her death.

A NEW JOURNEY IN MEDICINE

After Beth's death, I was ready to take a break from surgery.

In medical school, students spend a period of time rotating through each major medical specialty, supervised by resident and attending physicians. I began my next rotation in physical medicine and rehabilitation (PM&R), also called physiatry. This rotation intrigued me, as it took a different approach to musculoskeletal issues and care. Physiatrists or rehabilitation physicians have broad training in medicine, neurology, and orthopedics. We tend to emphasize using nonsurgical treatments to manage patients with a wide variety of neurologic and musculoskeletal conditions.

Gradually, I came to realize that physiatry was the specialty for me. I continued my training during my residency at the Mayo Clinic, where, unlike most hospitals at that time, the physiatry department was at the forefront of patient care. Patients who presented at the clinic with chronic lower back pain were first sent to see a physiatrist to obtain an accurate diagnosis and optimize their nonsurgical care, before considering any surgical intervention. In the rare circumstance that a patient needed surgery imminently, the physiatrist called in a spine surgeon to see the patient. What a commonsense approach: offer the least invasive treatment options first and give the body a chance to heal before intervening with more aggressive surgical treatments!

After my PM&R residency, I was fortunate enough to begin a sports medicine fellowship at the Hospital for Special Surgery (HSS) in New York. HSS was, and still is, an orthopedic surgery mecca. It boasts the best of the best orthopedic surgeons, not only in the country but in the world. As of 2022, HSS had been ranked number one in orthopedics for the past twelve consecutive years by U.S. News & World Report. When I started at HSS in the early 1990s, there was no physiatry department and I struggled to find my footing. However, I eventually found an excellent mentor in Dr. Russell Warren, who was a gifted, open-minded orthopedic surgeon, chief of sports medicine, and the team physician for the New York Giants.

After my fellowship at HSS ended, Dr. Warren hired me to improve the nonsurgical care of patients at HSS. A few years later, he became Surgeon-in-Chief and asked me to start and chair the first ever physiatry department at HSS in 1997. Looking back, without his support and vision, I do not know if HSS ever would have had a physiatry department. I was just thirty-five years old and chief of physiatry at HSS; my career path forward began to unfold in front of me.

To say it was a bit intimidating to start a brand-new physiatry department in this environment is an understatement. Although I was relatively young in my career, I was convinced early on that surgery was not the answer for most patients with CLBP. The problem I had at that point was that I just didn't know what to do with patients who did not respond to nonsurgical care. I saw how big a problem CLBP was, but I did not understand the underlying mechanisms that made the pain become chronic and resistant to standard treatments. Happily, I can report that, decades later, we have discovered a simple and safe treatment that I believe will transform how the medical field treats patients with CLBP.

THE HISTORY OF HSS

HSS, the oldest and one of the most prestigious ortho-pedic hospitals in the world, has a unique history. The hospital was founded by Dr. James Knight in 1863, in the middle of the American Civil War. At the time, hospitals were overwhelmed and unable to take care of children who were sick and suffering from orthopedic deformi-ties. In order to address the needs of those patients, Dr. Knight turned his home into a twenty-eight-bed hospital and called it the New York Society for the Relief of the Ruptured and Crippled.

In that era, given the frequency and severity of surgi-cal infections, few if any surgeries were performed during Dr. Knight's tenure. Most of Dr. Knight's patients received care in the form of exercise, bracing, and better nutrition—nonsurgical care. Things changed in 1887, however, when Dr. Virgil Gibney became Surgeon-in-Chief. He brought not only the first X-ray machine but also the first operat-ing room to HSS.

For the next hundred years, the hospital's focus shifted to providing surgical solutions for patients with orthopedic problems through patient care, research, and education. The name was later changed to Hospital for Special Surgery to reflect that focus.

> During the tenure of Dr. Russell F. Warren (Surgeon-in-Chief from 1993–2003) I was asked to start the first Physiatry Department of its kind in the country. I was Chief of Physiatry for fifteen years and built it into one of the largest outpatient interventional orthopedic practices in the country. Our mission was to provide orthopedic patients with state-of-the-art nonsurgical care. I like to think my efforts would have been pleasing to Dr. Knight by swinging the pendulum back to a more balanced approach to patient care.

*Sometimes inspiration comes from
the unlikeliest of places.*

As you can imagine, running a major department as a young physician was tremendously stressful. My days were long and included a regular commute from my home in Princeton, New Jersey, to New York City. "You need to slow down," my wife told me.

So I did, and we found a beautiful farm in Hopewell, New Jersey. We had always dreamed of raising our kids on a farm—and I reduced my time at HSS to four days a week. Those three days off at the farm were incredibly therapeutic for me. I would turn off the hospital stress and recharge, driving the tractor, fixing fences, and riding horses with my kids.

One day as I sat in the stable with a very skilled veterinarian, Dr. Daniel Keenan, as he tended to a lame horse, I had my "aha moment." Dan took a large amount of blood from the horse, spun it in a centrifuge to concentrate the cells, and then re-injected it, under ultrasound, into the horse's partially torn tendon. This was a new treatment at that time called **platelet-rich plasma** (**PRP**). Prior to this experience, I had never heard of PRP.

Historically, while anti-inflammatory medications, such as steroids, helped horses feel better temporarily, they were rarely a cure and often had to be repeated. Repeating steroid injections is a problem because it weakens the tendon, often leading to a complete rupture. PRP was different, and the results I saw were simply amazing. After the injections, our once-lame horse transformed in just a few weeks, running around the field like a young colt. And the most shocking part? The horse stayed better and never had to be injected again.

"You should be doing this on your patients," Dan said. I began to read the scientific literature on PRP. Interestingly, much of the science was coming out of the fields of dental and veterinary medicine, not orthopedics or physiatry. The more I read, the more I became intrigued with this emerging field of **regenerative medicine**.

As I watched our horse gallop happily across the field, I considered that, *just maybe*, this could work for my patients suffering from CLBP. The same collagen (Type I) that makes up tendons also makes up the outer fibrous rings of the discs in our spines. At that point in time, there were no published clinical studies on using PRP in the disc.

I immediately ordered a centrifuge and some PRP kits—the same kits Dr. Keenan had used on our horses. Because PRP is made up solely of the body's own cells and healing proteins, and not considered a drug, a full FDA trial at that time was not needed to begin to explore treating patients with this new therapy.

WHAT IS PLATELET-RICH PLASMA?

If you want to know the fascinating science behind how you can use your body's own cells to create healing, this section is for you.

Platelet-rich plasma (PRP) is a regenerative medi-cine treatment. It's autologous, meaning it's derived from your own blood. First, the blood is drawn, collected, and placed into a centrifuge to separate and concentrate the cellular components.

Spinning at that speed creates three distinct layers: blood plasma on top, the buffy coat that contains mainly platelets and white blood cells in the middle, and then the red blood cell layer on the bottom. The majority of red blood cells are then discarded, leaving the buffy coat full of plate-lets and white blood cells in the plasma. These are spun a second time to further concentrate them, creating PRP.

PRP contains a highly concentrated dose of your own healing platelets, with thousands of different proteins (growth factors) that promote wound healing and tissue regeneration. Platelets are not really cells but rather frag-ments of cells called megakaryocytes. Wherever PRP is placed, it simply ignites your own natural healing cascade.

The concept is pretty simple. When you suffer an injury to your skin and start bleeding, platelets are the first to the wound. They aggregate and form a clot to stop the bleeding. But that's not all they do; they then release a multitude of proteins called growth factors that signal waiting stem cells (called pericytes on your blood vessels) to come to the wound and begin the healing process.

Your body does this on its own beautifully wherever there is good blood flow to the area, such as the skin or muscle. The problem arises when you have an injury in an area with poor blood flow, such as a tendon, a spinal disc, or cartilage. In those areas, natural healing is often slow or incomplete. By injecting PRP precisely into these areas, you jump-start your own innate ability to heal—personalized medicine at its best.

PLATELET-RICH PLASMA

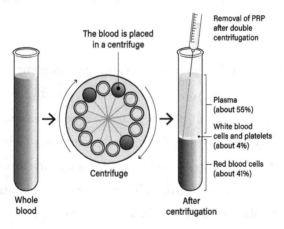

The blood is placed in a centrifuge

Centrifuge

Whole blood

Removal of PRP after double centrifugation

Plasma (about 55%)

White blood cells and platelets (about 4%)

Red blood cells (about 41%)

After centrifugation

Figure 1. This is how PRP is prepared. We draw your blood and place it into a centrifuge, and the cells of the blood are concentrated and separated into different layers. Erythrocytes are your red blood cells and go to the bottom of the tube. Then there is the buffy coat, which is composed of white blood cells and platelets. Plasma is the protein portion of the blood. We can now aspirate the concentrated platelets and white blood cells into the plasma to make the PRP to inject.

A NEW HOPE FOR PATIENTS

By chance, on the very first day my PRP kits arrived at my HSS office, a seventy-year-old patient, James, came hobbling in with a chronic tear in his Achilles tendon.

These PRP kits were one of the first to be commercially developed. They consisted of syringes to draw blood and containers to place into a centrifuge to spin the blood, which would then concentrate healing cells to about five times normal blood levels.

I knew that I did not want to begin experimenting by using PRP in the spine, which is a much more sensitive and risky area than a tendon. Based upon his injury and condition, James seemed like a possible candidate, but it was definitely a long shot. His injury was not a complete tear, but it was severe, roughly 70 percent torn, which would normally make him a surgical candidate. In pain and wanting to avoid surgery, he had been walking around in a boot for protection for six months with no signs of healing.

Coincidentally, as a hedge-fund manager, James had invested in a company making PRP kits, so he understood the technology and the research behind it. He'd gone to different orthopedic surgeons, and all had recommended surgery. When he came to me to explore the nonsurgical options, he asked, "Why is no one willing to try injecting PRP into my tendon? I came to you because I heard you might try this."

Now let me repeat: this was the very first day I received the PRP kits in my office. Here was a patient asking for PRP, and I was looking for a patient to try it on. Fate? Divine intervention? A coincidence? You can make your own judgment.

I made James no promises and certainly had significant doubts about it working, but what could be safer than using your own cells to potentially heal yourself?

Just to give some more perspective, in my busy sports medicine practice at HSS I had never seen an Achilles Tendon tear the size of James's ever heal on its own. I agreed with all the surgeons he had seen—he needed surgery. But I was willing to explore the PRP as an option because I knew it was safe.

I told him it was a definite long shot, but James was used to taking long shots in his hedge fund. He said, "It makes sense to me, so I'm game because I really would prefer to avoid surgery."

Carefully, we drew approximately sixty teaspoons of James's blood and spun it for fifteen minutes in a centrifuge, resulting in approximately five teaspoons of PRP. This very simple spinning method separates out the components of blood so that the heavier cells get layered out from the bottom up (red blood cells → white blood cells → platelets) and the plasma rises to the top (Figure 1).

Then, under sterile conditions and local anesthesia, I guided the needle under ultrasound precisely into the tear in James's Achilles tendon. As I injected the PRP, I could see that the tear was worse than what the MRI had shown. Nevertheless, I administered the treatment into the tear and surrounding areas. He experienced only mild discomfort afterward.

I sent James home and told him to return for a follow-up visit in a month. At his next visit, we both were pleasantly surprised. His pain was significantly better, but not 100 percent, so I performed a second PRP injection. When he returned a months later, his pain was gone, and he told me he had played tennis for the first time in over a year. "Not so fast," I said. "Let's see if the tendon is healed before you try tennis again." When we repeated the MRI (Figure 2), the Achilles tendon tear had healed completely. It looked completely normal! In all of my years of medical practice, I had never seen an injury like his heal without surgery.

He was ecstatic, and I was happily surprised.

You usually do not hit a home run with your first at bat, but that's what it felt like.

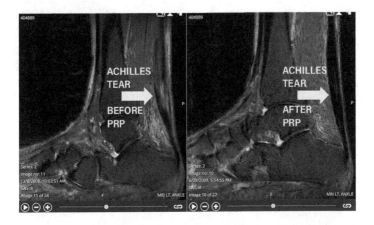

Figure 2. The MRI image on the left is a side view of James's left ankle showing a large tear of the Achilles tendon (arrow). The area of white inside the black tendon is the tear. The MRI image on the right is James's left ankle six months after his PRP injection showing a completely healed Achilles tendon (arrow). A normal tendon should look completely black on the MRI.

The skeptic in me thought, maybe this was a fluke?

So to prove the procedure's efficacy, we began injecting PRP into other patients with chronic tendon tears that had not responded to nonsurgical care. All of our tendon injections are done precisely under ultrasound imaging. What's so nice about this is that we can track healing with the ultrasound very simply in the office. It only takes a few minutes, unlike an MRI, which can take up to an hour and costs a great deal more than an ultrasound.

Previously, surgery had been the only thing left to offer such patients who had not responded to oral medication and physical therapy. Now, I wondered, what did they have to lose?

My surgical colleagues were very skeptical, and so was I at first—but one by one, the majority of our patients started to heal in just a few weeks. We achieved a high success rate, and other than some increased pain that resolved after the first few days, there were no complications.

> *Almost every patient was getting better.*

Those we'd have previously sent to months of physical therapy —and ultimately tendon surgery if that failed—were now getting better with a simple, thirty-minute outpatient procedure that used their own cells. Talk about personalized medicine; how much more personalized could it get?

I quickly realized that regenerative medicine using PRP and other cell therapies had the potential to change orthopedics as we knew it, offering new hope for patients seeking alternatives to surgery. The lingering question I had at this point was whether this treatment could have the same effect on patients with degenerative disc disease, which is the number one cause of CLBP.

What was also so encouraging is that not only were patients feeling better, but their ultrasound images were also showing structural changes in the tendon. Chronic tears were disappearing, and the tendon was looking normal again. Could PRP be just the answer I was searching for to help my CLBP patients? Afterall, most of these CLBP have painful tears in their discs—very similar to tears in tendons.

Could regenerative medicine hold the answer for your pain?

Yes, there is new hope for patients with CLBP, and it's not a new drug or a new type of surgery; it's turning inside and using your own healing cells, precisely guided to where they need to go with a simple outpatient injection procedure. Everything you need to heal is already inside of you. As you will learn, all it takes is a special type of PRP designed specifically for the inside of the disc, a type of PRP very similar to the one that healed James's Achilles tendon tear.

Are you struggling with chronic lower back pain?

You are not alone, and I am here to help you make better decisions about your spinecare based on my thirty years of clinical experience treating tens of thousands of patients with CLBP.

You will learn just how big a problem CLBP is not just in the United States but globally. It is another pandemic that we have not overcome with our current treatment strategies. The number of patients suffering from CLBP just keeps growing, and our current treatments often fall short of patient expectations.

Our traditional treatments of drugs and surgery are not root-cause treatments. These types of treatments are palliative at best. Instead of focusing on how to *cure* lower back pain, we have focused on suppressing the symptoms with steroid injections and opioids—or even cutting out discs and fusing the spine to try to get rid of the source of the pain.

Why are you in pain?

I'll help you uncover the answer and walk you through the reasons why:

- Painful unhealed tears inside your degenerating discs are the number one cause of CLBP.

- Bacteria play a greater role than we previously realized in degenerative disc disease and CLBP.

- Early intervention with a special kind of intradiscal PRP may be killing two birds with one stone (stimulating healing and killing bacteria).

To devise better solutions, we first need to better understand the underlying mechanisms that cause discs to degenerate. Only then can we devise treatment strategies that not only get to the root causes, but also prevent or reverse these degenerative processes to keep your spine healthy. The goal should be to heal without cutting and intervene early so that the spine does not degenerate into more severe deformities that create so much long-term pain and disability for patients.

What are my alternatives to spinal surgery?

My entire medical career, I have been searching for a better solution to treat CLBP than spinal surgery. After decades of looking for a safe solution, I think we have found one. It is not a drug or a surgery. It is your own innate capacity to heal using your own cells. No drug or surgery will ever mimic what the body already has evolved to do so well.

I will introduce you to this revolutionary new spinal procedure that we have researched and performed safely now for over ten years. It takes less than one hour, does not require any hospitalization, does not require general anesthesia, requires very little time off from work, is a fraction of the cost of spinal surgery, and carries significantly less risk than traditional surgical treatments. For most patients, this procedure is one and done; rarely does it have to be repeated, and if it does, it usually provides further improvement.

This information is too important not to share. There have been many promising treatments for CLBP that have come and gone over my career, but this one has staying power because it's a root-cause treatment. This procedure will shift the treatment paradigm of spinecare into the new field of regenerative medicine.

I will share with you real patient stories from my clinical

practices at one of the busiest orthopedic hospitals in the world and from my private clinic the Regenerative SportsCare Institute (RSI) in Manhattan. The patient names have been changed, but their stories and MRI images are real.

Are you a good potential candidate for regenerative medicine?

While regenerative treatments offer new hope for patients suffering from CLBP, they are not always successful and are not without risk. This field has been historically less regulated than other areas of medicine because it does not involve the use of a drug. This lack of regulation creates a confusing landscape for a patient with CLBP to try to navigate on their own. I will walk you through this decision making process step-by-step to ensure you protect your spine from ineffective and poorly conceived treatments.

I will educate you regarding what I feel is currently not only the most effective but also the safest regenerative treatment to consider. I will also give you some insights on how to find a reputable regenerative spine specialist to potentially treat you.

How will we make this paradigm shift toward regenerative medicine?

The way our healthcare system has managed CLBP is over-due for a radical change, but change is difficult. There are so many entrenched players in healthcare that can create barriers and resistance to change. For regenerative medi-cine to become mainstream, we will need to overcome them. I'll share my thoughts on a strategy that could work called vertical collaboration. It places the needs of the patient at the core and uses scientific evidence to make rational healthcare decisions.

I left the confines of a hospital to open RSI, further my research in regenerative medicine, and offer my patients this new treatment option in a more personalized environment. Unlike most hospitals, which focus on surgery, RSI's goal is to preserve the disc and spine with non-surgical care. Our primary focus is on finding a cure for lower back pain—the most common, the most disabling, and the most expensive musculoskeletal problem humans face. I feel the answer lies in healing painful tears in the discs early on in the disease process with nothing more than a special concentration of your own cells. What I have learned is that the needle is mightier than the scalpel when it comes to the treatment of CLBP, and your body is your best surgeon. If we can heal your disc, we can end your pain and hopefully halt or reverse degenerative disc disease.

In the next chapter, you will learn:

- Just how prevalent and costly CLBP is, not just in the United States but also globally

- How CLBP is a pandemic in its own right and how most treatments have been ineffective, causing too many patients to take long-term opioids or undergo needless spinal surgeries

- How the economic magnitude of this healthcare problem is staggering and a paradigm shift in its treatment is long overdue

CHAPTER 2

THE LOWER BACK PAIN PANDEMIC & THE OPIOID EPIDEMIC

"Most people who become addicted [to opioids] like me do so after a prescription for a painkiller following a medical procedure. Once the phenomenon of craving sets in, it is often too late."

—JAMIE LEE CURTIS

If we could choose a single nonfatal medical condition to find a better solution for that would make the greatest impact on global health, it would be a cure for degenerative disc disease (DDD)—the number one cause of CLBP.

According to the numbers, lower back pain is a pandemic— a condition that is prevalent globally, affecting millions of people around the world. In 2017, the Global Burden of Disease (GBD) Study reported that the point prevalence (the number of people in the world at one point in time) of activity-limiting lower back pain is about **580 million people worldwide**—and chronic lower back pain is now regarded as the number one cause of disability globally.[2]

This is the most comprehensive analysis of 354 medical conditions from 195 countries, for the nearly three decades between 1990 and 2017. Not only was CLBP the number one cause of years lived with disability (YLDs) recently, it has also been the number one cause every year since 1990—and its incidence is only increasing with time.

> *The numbers reported are staggering: as many as seventy million Americans have lower back pain today.*

An estimated 80 percent of all Americans will experience disabling lower back pain at some point in their lifetime. What was thought of as a benign condition, really is not. In my experience, many of my patients have chronic recurrent episodes of lower back pain that just keep getting worse over time. Frustrated, many physicians decide to prescribe pain medication because they do not know what else to do.

An epidemic is a condition that affects a large number of people within a region, and we have been dealing with an opioid epidemic here in the United States. Our mismanagement of LBP has only contributed to this problem; in the US, opioids are the most commonly prescribed drug class for patients with LBP, and the rate of opioid prescription is two to three times higher than in most European countries.[3] This practice occurs despite evidence that opioids, if used for managing LBP at all, should only be administered for acute pain and for a short duration of time (a few days at most).

> *Despite their widespread use, there is no research to support the long-term use of opioids for managing back pain.*

Complications of addiction and overdose have risen in parallel with increased prescription rates for LBP. According to the CDC, between 1999 and 2020, nearly 565,000 people died from opioid overdose involving both illicit and prescription uses.[4]

Anyone taking opioids can quickly become addicted—within weeks of daily use. More than 11.5 million Americans reported misusing prescription opioids in 2016.[5] Unfortunately, this trend has only increased; in 2021, overdose deaths from opioids increased to over one hundred thousand from both illicit and prescription-based causes. We are in desperate need of treatment alternatives to opioids for patients with back pain.

I commonly see CLBP patients who have had lumbar fusion surgery. Many of these patients had never taken opioids but were prescribed them at the time of their surgery to manage their post-operative pain. Even when opioids fail to provide adequate pain relief post-operatively, doctors often renew opioid prescriptions month after month. In a recent meta-analysis of patients after lumbar fusion surgery, investigators found that up to 63 percent of these patients were on long-term opioids (a duration greater than three months).[6]

This study also showed that opioid-naive patients (meaning patients that were not on opioids prior to their surgery), were at increased risk for long-term opioid use after their fusion surgery. Equally concerning is the fact that, despite these poor outcomes, one study found a 276 percent increase in the number of these types of lumbar fusions for degenerative conditions between 2002 and 2014.[7] What is driving this epidemic?

The results of lumbar fusion surgery are even worse in patients who were "injured" at work.[8] In a large study of Ohio worker's compensation patients with CLBP they compared the outcomes of those workers who underwent lumbar fusions (LF) versus those treated nonsurgically (controls) over a two-year period. These were previously healthy, on average thirty-nine-year-old patients (725 lumbar fusion patients versus 725 controls) who had injured their backs.

The majority had an injury to one or more lumbar discs. What these researchers found was that 76 percent of LF patients were still on long-term opioids post-surgery, 41 percent had an increase in the opioid usage after surgery, 36 percent had surgical complications, 27 percent required reoperation, and only 26 percent ever returned to work (RTW) compared to 67 percent of the controls.

Think about the millions of people suffering from back pain who then become dependent on opioids because their treatment was mismanaged with ineffectual, nonsurgical treatments or potentially made worse with spinal surgery. Drugs and surgery have not been the cure we have been seeking for the majority of patients with back pain. The economic consequences are not just significant for the individual who fails to get back to gainful employment, but also for our healthcare system as a whole. This approach has resulted in a waste of precious healthcare resources for our country that could be better used. In 2011, the respected Institute of Medicine

(IOM), now called the National Academy of Medicine, estimated that in the US alone, the total direct and indirect costs of chronic pain from musculoskeletal conditions to our economy ranged between $560 and $635 billion annually.[9]

Unfortunately, there has been low investment in research to find a cure for back pain because, as most people do not die from it, many are unaware of its severity. That is a gross miscalculation if you take into consideration the contribution of CLBP to prescription opioid deaths or the perioperative mortality rate—on average 0.2 percent—for lumbar fusion surgeries.[10]

The US National Institute of Health budget for research on cardiovascular diseases and cancer is dramatically larger than its budget for musculoskeletal conditions ($8.6 billion combined versus only $754 million in 2018). In 2016, musculoskeletal disorders were the largest health expenditures in the US at $380 billion.[11] *We spend more money treating musculoskeletal conditions than heart disease, diabetes, or cancer, but less than 10 percent of our research dollars are allocated to finding better treatments or a cure for them*.

The economic consequences of this misguided strategy are significant not just for the US, but for other countries around the world. The increased burden of nonfatal diseases such as CLBP on healthcare systems worldwide are posing considerable challenges to all healthcare systems not equipped to care for such complex and expensive conditions. While healthcare systems have made advancements in the management of fatal diseases, we have not made meaningful advancements in managing "nonfatal" conditions such as CLBP.

Just looking at these facts, we are able to deduce that CLBP is a serious ailment that we have not yet "fixed." So why not take a different approach to the problem? We need to reframe our thinking about the root causes of chronic back pain and target our treatments directly at them if we want to truly find a cure. We need simple, safe, cost-effective, scalable treatments that are durable in their effect, not treatments that temporarily address your symptoms or might even make you worse.

Evidently, the situation seems to be worsening. North Carolina researchers published a study in the *Archives of Internal Medicine* that found that the prevalence of lower back pain **doubled** over a fourteen-year period from 1992-2006. That's a startling finding. It has been estimated that approximately one quarter of adults in the United States reported back pain for at least one day in the past three months.[12]

So, what's behind the rise in back pain?

There is not one cause but several. Contributing lifestyle factors are smoking, obesity, too little exercise, and sitting way too much. Even too much exercise of the wrong kind could lead to back pain for some patients we see.

More people today are overweight than ever before. In fact, the World Health Organization (WHO) has coined a new term for this **globesity** (the global obesity epidemic). The United States is the leader of the pack when it comes to globesity, with an estimated 42 percent of Americans being overweight.

In the last thirty years, obesity has risen dramatically, along with more sedentary, technology-reliant jobs. There is no debate about the deleterious effects of sitting on not only our overall but in particular our spine health. The average American sits for ten hours per day. We sit for breakfast, we sit for our commutes, we sit in front of our computers for work, we sit for dinner, and then we sit for our entertainment in front of our TVs in the evening.

Our bodies were designed to move, not sit for hour after hour. The disc receives its nutrition through cycles of compression and relaxation, not the type of chronic compression that is generated when we sit all the time. This combined with the added pounds of pressure from being overweight causes the disc to begin to weaken prematurely.

Think of the disc as a radial tire with a gelatinous core that is surrounded by ten to twenty concentric fibrous rings whose job it is to keep that gel from leaking. Those rings are made of the same collagen that composes your tendons, but rather than being arranged in a linear fashion they are arranged in circles. The outer rings of the disc are called the **annulus fibrosus**, and the center of the disc is called the **nucleus pulposus** (Figure 3).

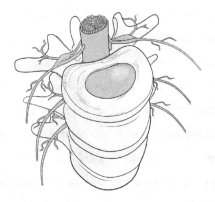

Figure 3. This is an illustration of the anatomy of the lumbar spine. The intervertebral disc is sandwiched between the bones in the spine called the vertebral bodies. The gelatinous center of the disc is called the nucleus pulposus. This is contained by circular rings called the annulus fibrosus. The spinal nerves rest in the spinal canal behind the disc.

THE INTERVERTEBRAL DISC:
A FLAWED STRUCTURE?

There's an annulus fibrosis which is the tough fibrous exterior of the intervertebral disc. It is sort of like a circular tendon. Then there's the nucleus pulposus, which is the soft inner core with a gelatinous material. The annulus fibrosus protects the nucleus pulposus, helping to keep the gel from herniating and leaking out into the nerve canal.

When the nucleus pulposus is intact, the gelatinous material is contained, and therefore, the spinal segment maintains its height and alignment. But when there's a tear, the gel leaks out like a chemical spill, creating severe inflammation. If enough herniates through it also can create nerve compression and injury.

Unfortunately, the annulus fibrosus is also one of the most richly innervated structures in the body. So, it's a terrible combination: you have a gel that incites inflammation when it leaks into an area full of nerves.

The inside of the disc has a poor blood supply. Its blood supply is limited to the outer annulus fibrosus. So when it tears, it doesn't heal very well, because the cells that do the healing just don't get there.

Think of the disc as a structure that is composed of a circular tendon that surrounds a gelatinous core. When the stresses generated in the rings of collagen exceed its inherent capacity from an acute injury or chronic overload (a fall, a sports injury, a motor vehicle accident, or excessive sitting), the disc can develop internal tears. Since there are typically no nerve endings inside the disc (only on the periphery), you would usually not feel the beginnings of these tears until they extend to the periphery. So for many of us, back pain is silent for a while, and then when it comes on it can be crippling.

Another subset of patients we commonly see in our practice are the "gym rats"—bodybuilders, powerlifters, and athletes who overexert their bodies in the weight room, with heavy loads and poor form causing excess stress to their spines. We frequently see deadlifting and power-squat injuries. The problem is that as your muscles get stronger you can maneuver heavier and heavier loads to the point that eventually something gives. In many cases, it's the disc in your spine that develops a tear inside because of the extreme compressive loads. Many athletes I see get injured more in the weight room than in their actual athletic activities. That is why working with physical therapists who are knowledgeable about spine safe exercise and proper biomechanics is an integral component of any spine rehabilitation program.

*The pandemic of 2020-2021 has only
fueled this rise in back pain.*

As gyms and fitness centers were closed, many of us were unable to exercise. We spent more time sitting in front of electronic devices, scrolling our lives away. The added stress and anxiety created by the pandemic only lowered our threshold to perceive our pain.

The back pain patients I see tell familiar stories: "I lifted the sofa and felt a tearing sensation; I swung the golf club and felt the shooting pain; I bent over to pick something off the floor awkwardly and felt a pop." They remember the episode vividly because when it comes on it can be very intense and frightening. Back pain can bring you to your knees, but what led up to that episode? We call them the proverbial "weekend warriors"—they spend forty to fifty hours a week sitting behind a desk, at a computer, and then suddenly expect their bodies to perform rigorous physical activity when the weekend rolls around and they want to hit a three-hundred-yard drive.

Smokers have a higher incidence of back pain.

As for smoking itself, there is scientific evidence that there is a causal link between smoking and back pain.[13] In fact, Stanford University researchers found in a survey of over 2,300 adults that smokers had a statistically significant higher level of reported pain in all areas of the body but especially pain in the spine. There is also evidence of a dose-response relationship between the number of cigarettes per day and back pain. So if you can't quit, at least cut back.

Not only is there a greater incidence of back pain in smokers, but smokers have worse pain that persists for a longer duration than non-smokers. This may be related to nicotine. Nicotine is a known constrictor of blood vessels. As you will learn, the disc already has a very tenuous blood supply, so when it tears and you are smoking, you are only impeding your chances to heal. It's already hard enough to get your healing cells inside the disc; smoking just aggravates the problem further.

In addition, there is strong evidence to suggest that smoking can adversely affect platelet function.[14] As you will learn in the coming chapters, this will affect your ability to heal after an injury to your disc. The combination of decreasing blood flow and inhibiting normal platelet function is a recipe for developing chronic back pain—just another reason to quit or cut back on your smoking.

To some degree, we are simply outliving our spines.

The pace of aging is much faster than in the past. According to the WHO, over the next couple of decades the proportion of the world's population over sixty years of age will nearly double, from 12 percent to 22 percent. The number of people aged sixty years and older outnumbers children younger than five years. While advances in medicine have enabled us to live longer, these same advancements have not found their way into keeping our spines healthy as we age. All countries face major healthcare challenges to meet the clinical demands of this demographic shift. Drugs and surgery have not met this challenge, but regenerative medicine can be a sustainable solution.

Many of the patients who come grimacing through my doors have gained excess weight as they have aged, coupled with the fact that they have become increasingly deconditioned due to their sedentary lifestyle. Once pain starts, it becomes a vicious downward cycle for many people. The pain inhibits their activities further, leading to a drop in muscle tone and poor posture. They start taking Advil like candy. This habit might help their pain only temporarily, so they start searching for solutions in all the wrong places.

Frustrated with their lack of improvement, they seek surgeons to "fix" them, only to go through an invasive spinal surgery that doesn't deliver the pain relief they expected and, in some cases, makes them worse. This only increases their anxiety and the intensity of their pain! I've seen this story play out so many times, unfortunately.

Remember James from Chapter 1? Let me share with you his full story as an example of what I am talking about. Once James's Achilles tendon was healed, he was anxious to get back to tennis. Within a few weeks of playing tennis, he developed severe back pain from a herniated disc.

> *It's not unlike the story of the typical "weekend warrior" we commonly see.*

James spent six months walking in a boot trying to protect his Achilles tendon tear, remaining relatively inactive. Before James's injury he loved playing tennis, and he often talked to me about how much he missed the game while dealing with his Achilles tear. Naturally, when James healed his Achilles with PRP, he quickly hit the courts—a little too quickly if you remember. And just as quickly he herniated a disc in his lower back. All those months of inactivity had caught up with him.

When James arrived at my office that Monday morning, he was understandably frustrated and unwilling to accept my recommendations to try nonsurgical care for his disc herniation. This would typically be an epidural steroid injection to reduce the pain and inflammation, followed by some physical therapy to build up his spine core muscles. If that didn't provide relief, we would then explore regenerative medicine options prior to considering any spinal surgery.

James wanted no part of it. "No way! I can't wait that long," he pushed. "I've waited for months already; I want my life back." James wanted that quick "fix." So, rather than take the conservative more patient path, James found himself a surgeon willing to perform surgery, where they made an incision and cut out the piece of disc putting pressure on his nerve. Initially, the surgery seemed to be a success.

But James's results were short lived: within weeks, more disc material extruded from the same level. This unfortunately is not an uncommon scenario. When surgeons remove a herniated disc, all they are doing is removing the disc material in the spinal canal that is compressing the spinal nerves. There is no reliable surgical technique that repairs the tears in the disc that led to the herniation. So that defect in the annulus fibrosus persists.

Surgeons have tried for years to suture it or use other methods, unsuccessfully. You hope the tear in the annulus fibrosus heals itself by scarring down, but it's an unpredictable process. It's called a **recurrent disc herniation** and can occur after this type of surgery, called a discectomy, in about 10–20 percent of patients.

> *Just because you have surgery to remove a disc herniation, it doesn't mean the disc is normal again.*

Most patients don't understand this—they think they are "fixed." James's pain was severe. So once again, he decided to return to the surgeon to cut out the extruded disc material (recurrent herniation) that was compressing his nerve. Each time you have surgery, the risk for infection goes up. The spine, and specifically the disc, have a unique "microbiome," (something you will learn more about in the coming chapters) that can make you more prone to developing an infection.

Unfortunately, James developed a very bad infection after his second surgery. He spent weeks in the hospital, flat on his back, struggling to recover while receiving high-dose antibiotics. For me, it brought back awful memories of what had happened to Beth; I hated seeing him suffer and feared the worst.

Nowadays, doctors are much more conscious of the deleterious effects that prolonged immobilization can have on the body, and therefore, take many more precautions to prevent the type of blood clots that killed Beth. Doctors put patients on anticoagulant medication, apply compressive boots on their legs to pump the blood out of them, and prescribe physical therapy early to get patients moving as soon as possible.

Thankfully James did not develop any blood clots, but once the infection cleared, James's spine now needed to be fused because the disc was destroyed by the infection. So he went back and had a third surgery—in just three months. This time it was a spinal fusion that involved placing screws and connecting rods to stabilize the spine and reduce the pain.

Afterwards, James could barely walk and had to use a walker everywhere he went. He needed chronic opioids to get through basic day-to-day tasks. He told me that his hedge fund lost millions of dollars because he couldn't concentrate after all he had been through. He also shared with me that he wished in retrospect that he had tried the more conservative approach I had offered him initially.

After about a year, he finally recovered and was able to walk without the use of a walker. But James would never return to his pre-surgery condition; he never went back to playing the tennis he so enjoyed. Shortly after James finally recovered from his spinal fusion, he developed cancer and died. I strongly believe that all the stress of the surgeries and the chronic pain played an indirect role in his demise.

I share James's story as an example because you need to know what clinical experiences have shaped my philosophy of patient care and why I am so motivated to find better solutions for my patients suffering from CLBP. I work with some of the best spine surgeons in the world at HSS for whom I have tremendous respect. They often do remarkable surgeries for my patients with severe spinal deformities or unstable spinal fractures. However, even most of them would admit that you should try the least invasive treatment approaches first before considering spinal surgery for back pain from DDD. Give yourself a chance to heal on your own, or with regenerative medicine. If for whatever reason you do not respond, surgery could always be reconsidered after all reasonable nonsurgical options have been tried.

On the surface, regenerative treatments may appear to take more time. Instead of a quick "fix," I tell my patients it is a slow incremental heal, usually a four- to eight-week process. You really do not want to alter the normal healing process by trying to speed it up. There is a natural healing cadence that has to occur for tissue to become strong again. Patients are under the misconception that if they go the surgery route, it'll be a quick fix that is permanent. Occasionally that is the case, but more often that's not the typical scenario. Even with most surgeries it takes as long to heal if not longer.

Patience is a virtue in medicine.

You constantly have to weigh the risk/reward with any treatment, whether it's non-surgical or surgical. While doctors try their best, we are not perfect and can make mistakes in both diagnosis and treatment. However, in this area of medicine these mistakes are amplified because so much is at stake when caring for someone's spine. It's more prescient to accept incremental improvements in your back pain with nonsurgical treatments than to opt for more risky surgical solutions because you want that quick "fix."

I can certainly understand the impatience and anxiety of patients like James. When you are in severe pain, your body is in the proverbial "fight-or-flight" mode. Patients are afraid that their body will stay broken forever. So, at the first promise of relief, they jump to be fixed. While there are certain circumstances that could constitute a true surgical emergency (cauda equina syndrome), the chances for this are extremely rare.

WHAT IS CAUDA EQUINA SYNDROME?

This information is not to scare you but rather to reassure you. Cauda equina syndrome can occur if there is severe acute compression of the nerves in the spinal canal from a variety of causes. Most commonly it is a large disc herniation, but there are also other causes like bleeding, infection, or a tumor.

When this occurs a patient might experience a combination of symptoms:

- Leg weakness
- Leg numbness
- "Saddle anesthesia" (numbness around your genital area)
- Bowel or bladder problems (such as incontinence or retention)

If you experience a combination of these symptoms, it is important to seek medical attention early. Once the diagnosis is confirmed by a thorough history, physical examination, and appropriate imaging studies, surgery to relieve the spinal nerve pressure gives a patient the best chance for a full recovery.

Thankfully this condition is extremely rare. It has been estimated to occur in only one in sixty-five thousand patients with lower back pain. That is in keeping with my clinical experience. I have only seen this occur twice over my thirty years of clinical practice, both times from a very large disc herniation, and both patients responded very well to surgical removal of the extruded disc.

Part of being a caring healthcare provider is setting up clear expectations for your patients from the start.

My hope with this book is to enlighten you about safer emerging regenerative medicine options before considering spinal surgery. In the next chapter you will learn:

- That back pain is a symptom and not a diagnosis

- That there are many causes of back pain and your first goal with your physician is to obtain an accurate diagnosis

- That my practice philosophy that has worked well for the past thirty years has been: **be aggressive with diagnosis and conservative with treatment**

CHAPTER 3

THE IMPORTANCE OF AN ACCURATE DIAGNOSIS

"Above all things, let me urge upon you the absolute necessity of careful examinations for the purpose of diagnosis. My own experience has been that the public will forgive you an error in treatment more readily than one in diagnosis, and I fully believe that more than one-half of failures in diagnosis are due to hasty and unmethodic examinations."

—**DR. WILLIAM MAYO**, 1861–1939

Most healthcare systems are designed to treat the patient's symptoms, rather than to diagnose and treat the root causes. What we need is not better fusion devices or "pain-management" programs—it is to find an actual cure for the most common causes of back pain. More attention needs to be placed toward prevention and early intervention with healing regenerative treatments to preserve your spine.

Drugs to relieve pain or surgery to cut your herniated discs out are simply not a cure; they are palliative at best. These treatments often fall short of patients' expectations and often have side effects. In many cases, patients have been misdiagnosed and mismanaged, and precious healthcare resources have been wasted with ineffectual treatments.

Sure, some patients have been helped by these treatments, but too often it is not enough for them to return to their previous level of activity. These therapies may have helped them out of the acute pain, but did it really cure them so they could return to activities with a restored and rejuvenated spine that did not degenerate over time?

Many patients, unfortunately, are rightfully scared of undergoing spinal surgery and just end up modifying their activities to avoid the pain. Their spines just continue to degenerate often leading to more severe problems. Many patients succumb to chronic opioid use just to numb their pain temporarily. We can do better than that, but first we need to obtain an accurate diagnosis of the root cause of your back pain.

We need to get to the root
cause of your back pain.

The diagnosis is more than half the battle with managing any patient with back pain. While there are many potential pain generators in the spine, by far the most common source is a problem with a disc. Let me share Jennifer's story as an example of the importance of how an accurate diagnosis is the first step in finding a cure for back pain.

One day, Jennifer, a twenty-year-old former college student, stepped into my office with her distraught mom. She had been referred to me by another physician for a second opinion because she was not getting better with her current treatments. As I sat and listened to her symptoms, I recognized the pain journey she described as one I've heard many times before. Jennifer suffered from severe, disabling back pain that had lasted for over a year. This is extremely unusual for someone so young.

The pain was so bad that she had dropped out of college and was taking Percocet around the clock just to get through her day; her life was miserable, and none of her previous treatments had made any improvement in her symptoms.

She had seen another specialist (a rheumatologist) before me and was given a presumed diagnosis of **Ankylosing Spondylitis (AS)**. AS is an autoimmune systemic disease which causes an inflammatory arthritis that affects the spine and usually starts in the joints of your pelvis (sacroiliac joints). Typically AS patients experience pain that is nearly constant and not positional—what we typically refer to as "non-mechanical" pain (not related to changes in positions of sitting, standing, or walking).

It can be worse at night and then associated with prolonged stiffness in the morning. Patients feel very stiff and start to slump forward. Sometimes it's also associated with other systemic symptoms like abdominal pain and diarrhea. There is a blood test which may be positive in patients with AS called HLA-B27 antigen test.

While she was HLA-B27 positive, this did not mean that her current symptoms were from AS. Not all patients with a positive HLA-B27 go on to develop AS. As I listened, it became clear to me that her pain was positional or what is called "mechanical" pain. This would suggest it was more of a musculoskeletal problem, not a systemic disease. Jennifer described the pain as unbearable whenever she sat upright and told me that the only time she got relief was when she would lie down and unload her spine with her knees flexed.

She was able to sleep once she found a comfortable position and did experience some morning stiffness, but it resolved quickly. In patients with AS, the stiffness typically takes longer —an hour or two to improve in the morning.

The pain would also radiate down both of her legs in certain positions such as when sitting and driving. These were more nerve-like symptoms, not something we would typically see with AS but rather with a problem with a disc in the spine.

> *As I listened to her, her previous diagnosis*
> *did not seem to fit her symptoms.*

One of the first things I try to assess when I'm listening to a new patient in the office is the question of whether their pain is mechanical or non-mechanical. I want to make sure I do not miss or delay the diagnosis of the other diseases that can present as lower back pain; what we refer to as the "red flags": tumors, infections, systemic inflammatory diseases, kidney stones, ulcers, aneurysms, and so on—the kinds of things that might kill you if missed but represent less than 1 percent of all causes of back pain.

Typically, pain from non-mechanical sources like those I just listed are constant, progressive, and not positional. The pain can present with systemic symptoms like fever, chills, night pain, night sweats, weight loss, or blood in your stool. Non-mechanical lower back pain is usually what we refer to as "crescendo" pain. It usually just keeps getting worse and worse over time until a diagnosis is made and the appropriate medical treatment is provided. It is important to get this question out of the way up front, so I just listen for clues as to whether there are any non-mechanical symptoms.

Mechanical lower back pain, on the other hand, while it can be severe, usually can be reduced by certain body positions. The causes of mechanical lower back pain are varied and can include musculoskeletal problems with discs, bones, joints, muscles, fascia, and the ligaments of the spine.

There is usually one primary area or root cause, but in many patients, as their spines degenerate a combination of different spinal structures can be involved. These spinal structures all have nerve endings to transmit pain, so they can hurt. As with Jennifer's pain, it is usually positional, which means it is more mechanical than non-mechanical.

Determining the source of pain is an important first distinction. As I examined Jennifer, I was thinking, "Okay, based upon how she describes her pain, it sounds so mechanical. It doesn't really seem to fit the diagnosis of AS." Plus, she was not responding at all to the treatments she was receiving for this presumed diagnosis.

As part of Jennifer's care, she had already had an MRI of her sacroiliac joints which, like her clinical description, did not support her diagnosis. In patients with AS, the MRI should show some inflammatory changes first in the sacroiliac joints, which connect the pelvis to the lowest part of the spine. Jennifer's MRI images showed none of the typical findings you see in AS. In fact, they looked normal to me.

In addition to suffering from pain for over a year with no improvement whatsoever, Jennifer was taking a powerful chemotherapy drug—Humira—to treat the suspected autoimmune disease. This drug carries with it the risk of suppressing your immune system, which increases your risk for developing cancer and infections. Obviously, this was a very aggressive treatment protocol for a twenty year old with a questionable diagnosis of AS, but she was nevertheless in severe pain, and her physicians were trying to help her. I did not immediately tell Jennifer my suspicions—that she had been misdiagnosed all along.

*It was now time for me to ask a few questions,
so I probed further into her history.*

"Jennifer, have you ever had any history of trauma to your spine?" I asked after listening to her at length.

"Yes," she said emphatically. "I was in a car accident about three months before my pain started. I was rear-ended while driving. But I did not have any immediate pain right after the accident. Do you think it might be related?"

I've seen this type of delayed pain after trauma before. The force of the crash can cause tears inside the disc that can fester and then progress over time if it does not heal on its own. Therefore, you may not feel any pain right away, but weeks or months later, as the tear inside the disc propagates, pain develops. You keep going through life as usual because you are not yet feeling any pain. Then suddenly you bend over and twist to pick something up and BAM!, you feel a lightning bolt of pain.

*In fact, you may be reading these words,
and realizing this is exactly what has
happened to you.*

The reason you might not feel the pain right away is because, as you have learned, there are very few nerve endings inside the disc. Most of these nerve endings are located only on the periphery of the disc. So if you develop a tear inside of the disc, it has to extend to the periphery before you really begin to feel pain. As a result, it can take time before you start to feel pain after a traumatic event like a motor-vehicle accident or a bad fall.

Jennifer's MRI of her lower back actually had shown a small tear (called an annular fissure or annular tear) in the lowest disc in her spine (L5-S1). This MRI finding had been dismissed by her previous physicians because they could not believe that that small tear could create this degree of pain and disability for her.

Lower back pain is not in your head—it is most commonly coming from inside your disc.

However, I had seen this scenario before in similar patients with CLBP over the years that had been refractory to medical treatments.

This unfortunately is not an uncommon scenario that I encounter in my practice. Despite all the clinical evidence—

her positional pain and the MRI finding of a tear—her extremely well-trained rheumatologist treated her aggressively with systemic chemotherapy because they did not know what else to do for her.

"We should see if that tear in your L5-S1 disc could possibly be contributing to your pain," I suggested. I still wasn't disputing the AS diagnosis fully at this point, but it just didn't add up.

Over the years, I have found that spinal injections can be an extremely valuable tool in diagnosing the exact source of the pain, because I can target a suspected area of the spine—in this case, the L5-S1 disc—and inject medications directly at the suspected site to see if it provides any short-term pain relief.

If the patient feels better after the injection, then I know that I am closing in on an accurate diagnosis. If not, I try another potential spot in the spine. It's not frequently curative, but it's a great diagnostic tool. In Jennifer's case, the procedure I performed was called a caudal epidural steroid and anesthetic injection, which is a great injection to target the L5-S1 disc.

There are different ways of doing an epidural injection in the spine, but we have learned over the years that this approach reliably places the medication directly on the back of the lower lumbar discs, right between the outer rings of the torn disc and the spinal nerves that are transmitting the pain. We are not injecting into the nerves, just around them. This is what I did for Jennifer.

I was anxious to see Jennifer sitting up in the recovery room after the injection.

I wondered to myself: would she still be in debilitating pain? Just fifteen minutes later as I was walking by, she said, "My pain's gone!"

Now, if the original diagnosis of AS had been accurate, injecting around the L5-S1 disc would have done nothing for her. But Jennifer felt like a million bucks from the local anesthetic in the injection, at least temporarily. That disc tear that all of her previous physicians saw on the MRI and told her was nothing, was in fact something—in my opinion it was the root cause of her pain.

It was time to get to work helping Jennifer's torn disc to finally heal.

She had just spent a year of her life in pain and was now also dependent on opioids—another problem that needed to be dealt with, not by putting her in detox, but rather by treating the source of her pain successfully.

Because Jennifer's pain was so severe and had persisted for an entire year, we quickly moved to the regenerative medicine options you are going to learn more about in this book. She had already failed all of the usual conservative treatment options and had given it more than adequate time to heal on its own—and obviously, it had not. Her life was miserable, and we wanted to change that.

I injected her disc with a special concentration of her own healing cells, similar to the PRP I did for James's Achilles tendon tear (Figure 4). After just one injection and three months of healing, Jennifer was off all her opioid pain medications, had stopped the chemotherapy drug for her presumed AS, and had returned to college.

Her MRI showed healing of the tear in her L5-S1 disc that had given her over a year of severe pain (Figure 5). She has never received any other treatment for her CLBP, and it has been over five years now.

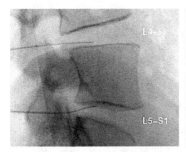
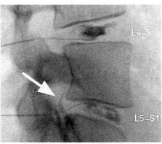

Figure 4. This is a fluoroscopic image (low dose X-ray) of Jennifer's injection into her discs of contrast (called a **discogram**). The images on the left are the needles placed into the two lower discs (L4-5 and L5-S1) without contrast injection. The images on the right are after contrast injection (black fluid inside the disc). In a normal discogram the contrast should stay in the center of the disc (the nucleus pulposus) and not leak out (L4-5 is normal). If you look closely at the lower disc, there is a faint black line of contrast (arrow) outlining the back of the disc that represents a tear of that disc (L5-S1). If the patient experiences similar pain to what they normally have (what is referred to as **concordant pain**) when we see the tear fill with contrast, then that is an abnormal discogram. The discogram helps us confirm the diagnosis of what is referred to as **internal disc disruption** when the MRI is inconclusive. We then injected PRP to trigger the healing response inside the disc to relieve her pain.

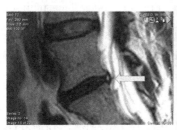
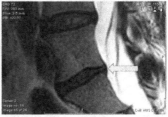

Figure 5. These are magnified MRI images of Jennifer's lumbar spine from a side view (sagittal views). The image on the left is before PRP treatment and shows a white line in the back of the disc (**called a high intensity zone [HIZ]**). The HIZ on the MRI represents a tear inside the disc. The image on the right shows the HIZ healed three months after PRP treatment.

*It was such a powerful and dramatic change
from such a simple and safe procedure.*

When she came back with her mother back for her three-month follow-up visit, she was a completely different person. It was a very emotional experience for everyone. To have so much pain and disability for so long relieved by a single injection of your own healing cells was profound. Fortunately we have helped many patients like Jennifer turn their life around with regenerative medicine.

As a physician, I strive to relieve a patient's pain and suffering. That is what gets me up in the morning to come to work, and that is what keeps me curious to find better solutions for my patients. There have been many potential promising treatments for patients with back pain that have come and gone over my many years of practice. The one you will learn about in the coming pages is different because it's a treatment that finally addresses the root cause of back pain—painful tears inside the disc.

Jennifer's story is an example of not only the importance of obtaining an accurate diagnosis, but also how regenerative medicine may be the CLBP solution we've been searching for.

Regardless of the source of your pain, if you're not getting an accurate diagnosis from the start, your chances of a cure are slim. An aggressive diagnosis, followed by a conservative treatment plan with an emphasis on regenerative treatments, is still your best approach in my experience.

In the next chapter, you will learn:

- More about how tears inside the disc are the most common cause of back pain

- Why these tears typically do not heal on their own and can lead to other more severe spinal problems that will necessitate spinal surgery

- Why the disc is the "heart" of the spine and our treatments should be focused on preserving it rather than cutting it out

CHAPTER 4

GETTING TO THE ROOT CAUSE OF DEGENERATIVE DISC DISEASE

"Gentlemen, I have a confession to make. Half of what we have taught you is in error, and furthermore we cannot tell you which half it is."

—DR. WILLIAM OSLER, 1849–1919

Our historic and current treatment paradigm for CLBP has been more about "putting the fire out" and trying to extinguish the pain symptoms with drugs or even trying to cut out the source of pain and replace it with screws, rods, and other implants. I tell my patients who are considering spinal surgery, "If you have a heart attack, they do not cut your heart out." They try to help the heart heal by restoring blood flow to damaged areas. So why are so many patients getting their discs cut out? We need to shift the spine treatment paradigm to trying to preserve the disc and help it heal early on in the process so that we can prevent more severe long-term problems. For those patients that present to our clinic with more advanced stages of disc degeneration that have led to a severe spinal deformity, spinal surgery may be necessary.

> *The earlier a disease is diagnosed,*
> *the easier it is to treat.*

You don't want any medical problem to persist and progress to later stages of disease, especially with conditions like cancer, for example. If we take this same approach with your spine, the ideal then is to quickly obtain an accurate diagnosis when you become symptomatic, followed by early intervention with regenerative medicine to heal the area of your spine. That is why we need to focus on root-cause treatments—to prevent injured discs from degenerating further.

Many patients with back pain are unfortunately in denial, hoping that their pain will miraculously disappear on its own.

They keep modifying their activities, hoping that time will help them heal on their own. As you have learned in the previous chapters, too often that is not the case. Many patients have justified fear over the risks of spinal surgery and turn to other, less risky treatment providers such as chiropractors, acupuncturists, physical therapists, and/or massage therapists.

> *Early intervention with regenerative medicine may limit long-term problems.*

Let's talk about disc herniations for example. There are different types of disc herniations (Figure 6).

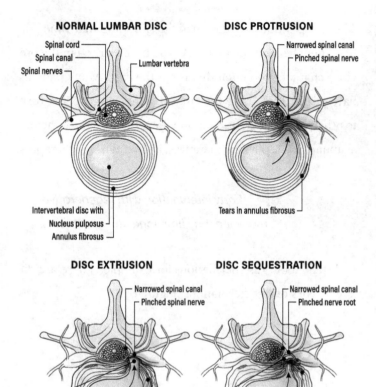

Figure 6. This is an illustration of the progression of a disc herniation from normal, to protruding (an incomplete tear), to an extrusion (a complete tear), to a sequestered disc (a fragment of disc material in the spinal canal), creating injury to the spinal nerve.

Types of Disc Herniation

- **Bulge:** This is when the outer layer of the disc, the annulus fibrosus, bulges out into the spinal canal, like a hamburger that's too big for its bun. Here, only the outer layer of the tough annulus fibrosus is involved.

- **Protrusion:** This is when a tear in the tough outer layers occurs, allowing some of the soft inner gel from the nucleus pulposus to escape into the nerve canal, like a pimple with a focal extension. Here the annulus fibrosus is still partly intact.

- **Extrusion:** This is when the annulus fibrosus is completely torn and the gelatinous material has herniated into the spinal canal, compressing and inflaming the nerves, like a chemical spill. However, it is still in contact with the mother disc it came from.

- **Sequestered Disc:** This is when a fragment breaks off from the main structure of the disc and is floating in the spinal canal.

It's rare to get a permanent nerve injury with just a disc bulge or protrusion. However, severe nerve injuries can occur when a disc extrudes its contents into the spinal canal and compresses a spinal nerve. Once a nerve is injured, recovery is long and often incomplete. So treatments that intervene early and can create healing of the tears inside the rings of the disc (annulus fibrosus) and shrink the protrusion before it pops will potentially prevent not only the need for spinal surgery but more severe and permanent nerve injuries.

These spinal nerves are important to protect because they control not only your ability to walk but also your bowel, bladder, and sexual function. That should get your attention!

That is why so many patients are turning toward regenerative medicine for a better solution to back pain. Early intervention with a healing treatment will hopefully prevent a disc protrusion from continuing on to a full extrusion or on to severe degeneration. These are two conditions that create more severe pain and disability for patients and may need more aggressive surgical intervention.

WHAT IF YOU JUST DO NOTHING?

In medical school, we were taught not to worry too much about lower back pain because in most patients it will get better on its own. In fact, on the patient's chart their diagnosis would often just say, "lower back pain." I found this confusing because "lower back pain" is a symptom, not a diagnosis.

There was very little diagnostic workup back then and very little conservative care. This was unlike any other area of medicine I was exposed to where an accurate diagnosis was critical to designing a successful treatment strategy. No wonder chronic back pain is so prevalent. The medical establishment has never given it the attention it deserves to really find root-cause treatments like intradiscal PRP. It was benign neglect—or so we thought.

Where's the data to support this hypothesis, that back pain's course is benign? There isn't any. In fact, the natural history of lower back pain is relatively unknown because frankly, it's been very hard to study.

It's difficult to capture enough patients who are experiencing a first-time episode to perform an accurate longitudinal study—everyone is at different stages, and everyone has different causes. It's such a mixed bag that needs to be better organized. The only way to accomplish this is to make an accurate diagnosis, categorize patients, and then follow them over time. Maybe with future advancements made in biomarkers, imaging, and artificial intelligence, we will make better progress on this issue.

In 2012, researchers published a study in *Physical Medicine and Rehabilitation* that tried to investigate this issue by surveying thirty different practitioners from a variety of specialties including physical therapists, chiropractors, and surgeons to look at the disease progression of CLBP in 589 new patients.[15]

Here's what these researchers found:

- Thirty-four percent said their back pain required more than three months to improve.

- Fifty-four percent reported more than ten episodes of severe, disabling back pain.

- Twenty percent reported more than fifty episodes of severe, disabling back pain.

My patient, Wendy, suffered from back pain for many years despite our best efforts at the time.

We treated her back pain conservatively with the standard course of oral medication and physical therapy. When that didn't work, we would administer an epidural steroid injection periodically to calm the pain and inflammation down so she could walk again.

The problem with this approach is that, while she would get temporary relief for a few months, each time the pain came back it got worse and worse. The pain that was originally in her back started to radiate down her legs until the point at which she developed weakness and could not walk more than a few blocks. What began as a small tear in her L4-5 disc never healed and eventually led to complete degeneration of that disc and progressive slippage of the spinal segment, and then to severe narrowing of her spinal canal with compression of her nerves (Figure 7).

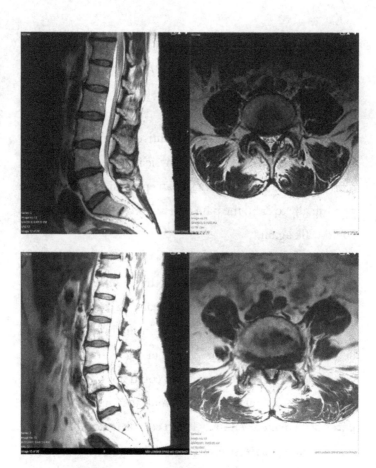

Figure 7. These are Wendy's MRI images of her lumbar spine over time. The top images are from 2013 when I first saw her, and the bottom images are from 2021. The MRI images on the left are looking at the spine from the side (sagittal T2), and the images on the right are cross-sectional images (axial T2). Note how the second from the lowest disc (L4-5) on the top view has a small tear and disc protrusion. The images on the bottom reveal the progression of disc degeneration over time with traditional conservative care. This resulted in narrowing of the spinal canal (stenosis), slippage of the spinal segment (spondylolisthesis), and led to her having major spine surgery to relieve her symptoms.

This is an example of what is referred to as the **"degenerative cascade"** that leads so many patients into a state of chronic pain and disability.[16] Unfortunately, it's a very real phenomenon that I have witnessed all too often. In its later stages, the joints of the spine can become large and arthritic because of the increased load placed on them now that the disc is deflated. This also happens to the ligaments of the spine, which can become thick and lax. This combination of events can lead to a narrowing of the spine called spinal stenosis. Some patients can also develop a spinal deformity: either a curvature (scoliosis) and/or a slippage (spondylolisthesis) of the spine. These are conditions where spinal surgery can be helpful to relieve the pressure on the spinal nerves and restore spinal alignment.

The degenerative cascade demonstrates the importance of acting early with root-cause treatments that heal the disc, so that this downward spiral can be avoided. As you can see, wound healing is a necessary and dynamic process for restoring the normal architecture and functionality of tissue; with disc tears, this process has gone awry.

It's really no different than when someone develops chest pain or **angina**. Angina is a condition of severe chest pain that can radiate into your left shoulder (the side of the body where the heart resides), back, and down the arm. Thankfully we have become acutely aware that this may be a signal of something worse like a heart attack. To intervene early with treatments that improve the blood flow to critical areas of the heart can save your life. To ignore these symptoms could lead to heart failure or even death.

That is the role of an interventional cardiologist—to precisely guide catheters and stents to reopen clogged blood vessels in your heart so that you do not die or reach those later irreversible stages of heart disease. Starting to see some of the similarities between interventional cardiology and interventional orthopedics?

Why have we not taken a similar approach when someone develops back pain? Why don't we get an MRI of the spine right away and see if there is a tear in a disc that we can treat before it goes on to a full-blown herniation that can permanently damage the nerves to your leg or your bowel and bladder function? The reason is because we never before had a root-cause treatment like you are going to learn about in this book.

The disc is the "heart" of the spine.

There is an emerging field of **interventional orthopedics** that is going to change how we manage back pain for the better. These like-minded physicians are already taking exactly that approach to back pain and combining it with advanced therapies from regenerative medicine to halt or reverse the dreaded degenerative cascade. My goal is to treat the disc like it is the heart of the spine and try to heal it so we can preserve your spine's function for as long as you live. Is this really possible?

> *Can we intervene early with back pain*
> *to halt or reverse degenerative*
> *disc disease?*

In medicine, there are times when you might be the first patient to try a new therapy. That's when I met Jeff, a forty-five-year-old financial advisor who came to see me after falling off a roof while trying to clean his gutters one weekend. Jeff could not sit without having severe back pain. Unfortunately, sitting is what he did for most of his workday. I wasn't his first physician; he'd been suffering for years by the time he came to my office to seek alternatives to a spinal fusion, which was what was recommended to him by a spine surgeon he saw.

Prior to our visit, Jeff had tried the standard conservative care: oral medications, epidural steroid injections, acupuncture, chiropractic care, and physical therapy. He said the only thing that helped him was the epidural injection, but it only gave him a few weeks of relief. Finally, in preparation for a spinal fusion, doctors had performed a test called a **discogram**.

A discogram is a test where a needle is inserted into your discs under fluoroscopic-guidance (low-dose X-ray), and contrast dye is then injected. In a normal disc without tears the contrast should stay in the middle of the disc (the nucleus pulposus) and look like a cotton ball on imaging. The patient might experience some pressure but usually not pain if it's normal. However, in a disc with a tear you will see it leak, sometimes all the way out of the disc and into the spinal canal. When this happens it may stimulate the patient's back pain.

What's most important with this test: does it reproduce your typical pain that limits you (**called concordant pain**)? Discography has a controversial history, but it was used in the past when the MRI was inconclusive and the surgeon wanted to make sure that if they were going to cut the disc out and fuse your spine, they were doing it at the correct levels. This was the case with Jeff.

I never enjoyed performing discograms, because I knew if it was abnormal the patient was going on to a spinal fusion. I would try everything reasonable with my patients to avoid that scenario. Unfortunately, back then we didn't have as many tools in our toolbox as we do now with regenerative medicine. While discograms have had a bad rap as a diagnostic test, the same technique coupled with injecting PRP can be an invaluable treatment option.

The frog has become a prince.

That discogram test I used to despise I am now excited to perform, because now, instead of just injecting contrast dye to diagnose whether the disc is the source of the pain, we can, at the same time, deliver healing cells and proteins precisely where they are needed to reduce or eliminate your back pain.

So instead of injecting two to three teaspoons of contrast dye into the disc, we now only inject maybe a half a teaspoon of dye to see the tears fill and then switch the syringe and inject at least two teaspoons of your PRP. As you will soon learn in the coming chapters, because of this discovery, very few of our patients go on to spinal fusion anymore.

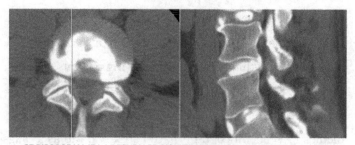

CT DISCOGRAM AT L4-5 REVEALED SIGNIFICANT ANNULAR DISRUPTION IN 2010

Figure 8. These are Jeff's CT Scan images of his discogram.
The images on the left are a cross sectional view (axial) from the
second lowest disc (L4-5) where we see the contrast dye (white)
leak out of the periphery of the disc (grey). The CT Scan images on
the right are a side view of the spine (sagittal) showing the
contrast dye leaking out of the back of the L4-5 disc.

When I looked at Jeff's CT discogram (Figure 8), it was bad. His discogram showed a blown-out disc from the impact of falling onto the ground from about ten feet up. The force had internally disrupted his disc, and he had two big tears, which meant Jeff was in pain because the gel from the nucleus was leaking into his spinal column, inflaming his nerves to no end. Jeff seemed like a potential candidate for my first intradiscal PRP procedure. His disc still wasn't fully degenerated, and while it was torn and bulging, there was still good height to the disc and no severe spinal nerve compression.

Since Jeff had failed all other treatments, I said, "We could try injecting into the disc some of your own healing stuff called platelet-rich plasma. I've recently had tremendous success treating tendon tears this way, but I've not tried it yet on the spine."

I made sure that Jeff knew that I had no idea if it would work but that I believed it was safe based on my review of the scientific literature and my experience with treating patients with tendon disorders. I felt confident that regardless of our success or failure, this would be much less risky than the spinal fusion he was otherwise fated to undergo.

I informed Jeff thoroughly on all the unknowns and the potential risks to the best of my knowledge; he knew that he'd be the first. "Sign me up!" said Jeff without hesitation. He was exhausted and tired of the chronic back pain and really did not want to get fused.

Once again, I really didn't know what to expect. At that time, while there was supportive preclinical data, no one had yet published a clinical study in humans. We were in uncharted waters, which in medicine can be exciting but also a nerve-racking place to be.

I worried about all the things that could potentially go wrong. However, in medicine, you have to judge the potential benefits versus the risks of your intervention, and you cannot let fear dictate your actions. In my medical opinion, the potential benefits for Jeff outweighed the potential risks, so we proceeded with the intradiscal injection of PRP. Other than some pain when we filled his disc with his PRP, the procedure went smoothly, and Jeff left hopeful that day.

When he returned weeks later, Jeff's outcome was considerably better than I had expected—just as with James's Achilles. At his eight-week follow-up, Jeff's lower back pain was almost completely gone, after years of suffering.

How long would this last? I continued to follow him, and the pain just kept getting better and better, month after month. Then I lost track of him and did not see him until eleven years later when he started to develop some recurrent back pain. He told me he had had eleven pain-free years after the PRP treatment and was able to go back to all of the sports he had enjoyed.

I was anxious to see what the treated disc looked like, so we repeated the MRI images of his spine to see if the disc had degenerated.

Unlike Wendy's story, Jeff's story was completely different. The disc we treated with PRP showed no signs of any degeneration at all. To the best of my knowledge, Jeff's case is the longest follow-up there is on any patient treated with intradiscal PRP.

Could PRP finally be the game changer we have been searching for in patients with chronic back pain?

2010   2021

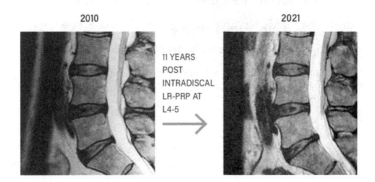

11 YEARS POST INTRADISCAL LR-PRP AT L4-5

Figure 9. These are Jeff's sagittal T2 MRI images. The MRI images on the left are from 2010, pre-treatment, and the images on the right are from 2021. There were no signs of disc degeneration at the L4-5 level over an eleven-year period post-PRP treatment.

Jeff's case is an example of the potential value of treating the root cause of back pain, which for most patients are painful unhealed tears inside the disc. Now that you have learned disc problems are the most common source of back pain, I will now explain in more detail new theories about the underlying mechanisms that lead to degenerative disc disease.

How many of you have been told that your back pain is just a strain of a muscle and should get better with time? "It's nothing to worry about."

Well, if you have ever torn a muscle elsewhere in your body you know that it might take a few weeks to feel better, but it usually heals just fine without any long-term problems. That's because muscles have an excellent blood supply and the human body has an amazing capacity to heal itself if the cells in the blood get there. So when muscles tear, the blood cells that do the healing are readily available and begin their repair work almost immediately.

Generally, when the injured tissues in the body have a robust blood supply, the chances of them healing are quite good. Look at what happens when you cut your skin; the wound quickly closes, and the skin tissue regenerates beautifully in most cases. Conversely, when the injured tissue has a poor blood supply—referred to as avascular—the chances of that structure healing on its own are poor.

A tendon is relatively avascular, and so are the discs in your spine. So when they develop tears, you get inflammation and pain but generally not healing. For example, prior to using PRP, a rotator cuff tear in your shoulder was difficult to heal without surgery. Many times it had to be surgically repaired, but no longer with regenerative medicine. We treat rotator cuff tears all the time now with regenerative medicine and have good success.

However, there is no reliable surgical technique to repair torn discs. This is because the collagen in the disc is arranged in multiple concentric layers, it is avascular, and it's difficult to unload. Your disc is almost always under tension, particularly when you sit, bend, or stand. The position with the least pressure on your disc is when you lie flat.

Plus, inside the center of the disc, there are potent proteins that incite inflammation when they leak outside of the disc. The analogy I give patients is that it is like a chemical spill onto the nerves in the spinal canal. The disc just stays inflamed and painful because the healing cells in your blood cannot penetrate inside the disc to create the necessary healing.

> *Chronic back pain is nothing more than an unhealed wound.*

Proper wound healing requires the migration of cells to the wound. Therein lies the root cause of a great deal of back pain that becomes chronic. It's nothing more than an **unhealed** *wound* inside a disc with a great deal of inflammatory proteins and nerve fibers that complicate the healing process. It's that simple.

The disc is one of the most pain-sensitive structures in the human body. When we start to view back pain as an "unhealed wound," you can see how it might change our approach to treatment.

How do your cells heal wounds?

Your blood cells heal wounds throughout your body in a three-phase process: blood clotting (hemostasis), inflammation and proliferation, and then remodeling (Figure 10). Platelets are not actually cells but rather cell fragments (from larger cells in the bone marrow called megakaryocytes). They are the key to initiate this process. They are the first to get to the wound and initiate the wound-healing cascade.

The inflammatory stage takes minutes to days to form. Let's say you cut your skin; the first platelets go to the cut where they mediate inflammation, aggregate, and create a clot. Then they release growth factors, which are signals to dormant stem cells that reside on the blood vessels (called pericytes) to wake up and migrate to the wound. White blood cells are also called in to attack bacteria that may have penetrated the wound to prevent an infection.

Now you're in the proliferation phase, which takes days to weeks. Here, those stem cells differentiate into the cell type needed by that tissue to create wound healing by laying down more collagen to regenerate the damaged tissue over time.

Finally there's the remodeling phase, which takes weeks to months, where the collagen hopefully matures back to normal as it is gently stressed with activities. The healing process is not a solo—it is a symphony of cells and proteins that have been designed to work together in synchrony with a pre-defined cadence. This process is unique to each one of us and is largely dictated by our genetic makeup—or our **genome**.

In the era of personalized medicine, there is nothing more personal than using your own cells to heal your disc.

The human genome is your complete genetic makeup: you come into the world with it. It is uniquely yours, and its code is written with 6.4 billion letters (nucleotides).

Everything you need to heal is already inside of you.

No worries, because you already have what you need inside you to heal. All we are doing with injecting PRP inside your disc is placing a high concentration of your specifically designed healing cells and proteins precisely where they are needed to relieve your back pain. So far in our research, the higher we can concentrate these cells and the more precisely we can place them in those painful tears, the better the outcomes.

WOUND HEALING

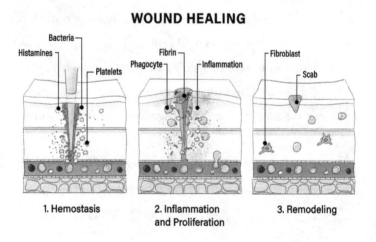

1. Hemostasis   2. Inflammation and Proliferation   3. Remodeling

Figure 10. Depicts the stages of normal wound healing.

The low blood supply to the disc is also why most medical and surgical treatments for back pain fail to provide sustained relief. They are not addressing the underlying root causes.

Yes, there are some patients that eventually improve without interventions, but this is most likely because some have a slightly better blood supply to the region and with time heal on their own or the size of the tear was small and had a chance to heal on its own. In general, the larger the tear, the harder it will be to heal on its own.

No one wants to find themselves in a degenerative cascade, so if you are not healing on your own after about eight to twelve weeks, I recommend exploring your regenerative medicine options. Specifically, when we intervene and use regenerative medicine, it brings a high concentration of those healing blood cells directly to the source of the injury and allows the tears inside the disc to heal.

We are injecting billions of platelets with thousands of different healing proteins into the disc tissue to stimulate this wound healing process. It can not only change a person's life in the short term but may also prevent the dreaded degenerative cascade that can happen if left untreated.

In the next chapter, you will learn:

- That like any unhealed wound it can become infected with bacteria

- That bacteria plays a larger role in back pain than we previously realized and we need to take this into account with our root-cause treatments

- Why infection has become the number one cause of spinal fusion failure

CHAPTER 5

THE ROLE BACTERIA PLAY IN DEGENERATIVE DISC DISEASE

"Gentlemen, it is the microbes who will have the last word."

—**DR. LOUIS PASTEUR**, 1822–1895

You may have heard the term microbiome as it relates to your gut, but what about in reference to your spine? A microbiome is an environment of trillions of microorganisms also called microbiota or microbes.[17] These can be a collection of thousands of different species of bacteria, fungi, parasites and/or viruses that live in harmony when you are healthy but are harmful when out of balance. This imbalance is referred to as "dysbiosis." Scientists are just realizing the importance of the microbiome not only for your overall health, but also with regards to your back pain.

The science of spinecare is constantly evolving; there's a whole new concept that the disc too has its own unique microbiome like the gut. A recent study out of Sweden looked at the role the intradiscal microbiome might play in degenerative disc disease.[18] The study examined 162 patients who experienced chronic lower back pain and had particular changes in their MRI (referred to as Modic Type 1 changes [MC1]). None of these patients had any history of any spinal surgery.

In a double-blind randomized controlled study (DB RCT), they separated the patients into two groups and gave one group a one-hundred-day course of oral antibiotics and the other group a placebo. The subset of patients that received the antibiotics improved to a greater degree than the control group. Their findings suggested bacteria may be playing a greater role in the back pain caused by degenerative disc disease than we had previously realized.

This issue was also studied from patients having spinal surgery where they harvested disc material, whether from a herniation or degeneration, and cultured that material to see if any bacteria would grow. Sure enough, study after study showed that bacteria grew on the disc material, and the most common bacteria was *C. Acnes*. At first investigators thought that this was from contamination, but that has later been refuted. The presence of *C. Acnes* infecting extruded and degenerative discs has been unequivocally demonstrated now by more sophisticated testing measures.

In 2016, a group of researchers in China actually took bacteria (*C. Acnes*) harvested from human-disc surgical samples and injected it into rabbit discs to see its effects.[19] When they examined the discs by MRI and under the microscope weeks later, these injected discs demonstrated exactly the same findings you see with degenerative disc disease and MC1 on MRI.

So why not treat CLBP patients with oral antibiotics? There are a number of valid reasons:

1. The lingering question of whether or not bacteria in the disc represents infection or contamination

2. Contradictory reports on the clinical efficacy of antibiotics to treat CLBP patients

3. The potential that widespread use of systemic antibiotics would result in emerging global

antimicrobial resistance, and the perceived risk of propagating superbugs

4. Systemic antibiotics that wipe out your gut's microbiome, creating other negative health consequences (patients in these studies had to take the antibiotic for one hundred days)

5. The unreliable penetration of most oral antibiotics that rely on blood flow to get to the disc

In another very recent study looking at the role of bacteria in degenerative disc disease, researchers took samples from healthy discs from patients with no history of CLBP or surgery and compared them with samples from patients with degenerative disc disease.[20] With sophisticated testing methods that look for the presence of bacterial DNA, they found that even healthy discs had a plethora of bacteria—there were 424 different bacterial DNA present!

This was the first study to show that even discs that appear normal on MRI have their own unique microbiome. When they looked at patients with degenerative disc disease, they found a dysbiosis, or an overgrowth of certain types of bacteria that weren't typically in normal discs.

What's so unique about this study is that it showed the presence of bacteria even in healthy discs without any external intervention. We always thought that the disc was a sterile environment, but apparently it is not. Think for a moment about the implications of this new finding as it relates to spinal surgery and the use of implants. Let me explain further.

THE INTRADISCAL MICROBIOME AND SPINAL FUSIONS

I only recently began to understand why some of my patients who had spinal fusions also had persistent pain after surgery for reasons that weren't clear. The x-rays of the spinal implants looked fine, but the patients were miserable and needed opioid pain medications just to get through their day. Why? New research suggests putting implants into a space that already has bacteria present is most likely the cause. We now know the spine is not a sterile environment.

If the primary cause of pain for some lower back pain patients is dysbiosis, then introducing spinal implants into this area will only exacerbate the problem. These implants act like a breeding ground for bacterial cells to attach and proliferate. What is equally concerning is that the number of these types of lumbar fusions with implants for degenerative conditions has increased 276 percent from 2002–2014.[21]

Wound studies of other orthopedic procedures with varying conditions have shown that the body has the capability to clear bacteria from the surgical wound rather well, except when there's an implant present. When you have an implant—a metallic surface—infections can occur much more easily, with far fewer bacteria present—one hundred to ten thousand times less.[22] It's a foreign body that provides a surface on to which bacteria can attach.

There's a well-known concept when surgically placing any medical device in the body: *the race to the surface*.[23] In the first few hours after an implant is surgically placed in the body, there is a race to the implant surface between normal cells and bacteria. If normal cells get there first, the implant is incorporated without difficulty; however, if bacteria win the race, then bad things can happen, like infection.

There are two main types of infections: acute systemic and chronic local. In an acute systemic infection, the patient develops symptoms of fever, chills, pain, abscess formation, and wound drainage shortly after surgery. Usually their blood work shows abnormalities like an elevated white blood cell count and elevated inflammatory proteins (an elevated sedimentation rate and an elevated C-reactive protein). In such cases, there is no doubt to you or your surgeon that there is an infection going on. Thankfully, this type of full-blown infection is rare, and that is why most surgeon's state their infection rate is only 1–2 percent.

However, that rate is misleading because it does not include the rate of chronic local infections (also referred to as delayed/occult infection) which are frequently underreported because they are very difficult to diagnose. With a chronic local infection of spinal implants for example, a patient does not usually have all of the obvious systemic signs of an infection and often their blood work is completely normal. The post-operative pain just never gets better and often worsens over time.

The reason is because these types of infections are associated with what is called biofilm.[24] Biofilms are layers of proteins on the surface of the implant produced by bacteria to protect them from the body's immune system and antibiotics. Think of biofilm as a bacterial protective force field from the body's immune system attack. The body is constantly attacking the biofilm with inflammatory white blood cells to no avail. It's like being stuck in the inflammatory stage of wound healing.

There is no reliable way for our bodies to clear infections from implants covered with biofilm. The only solution ultimately is to remove the implants all together. So what is the risk for delayed/occult infection with biofilm development on spinal implants?

As the world's experts in spinecare, my colleagues at HSS were quick to begin their own research. Dr. Frank Cammisa (a spine surgeon) and Dr. Celeste Abjornson (Director of Spinal Research) started studying the issue by culturing the spinal implants from patients with persistent pain after spinal fusions who returned to the operating room to have their hardware removed for a variety of reasons.[25] In their first study, they took cultures from the surface of the removed implants and found the presence of bacteria in over 40 percent of these patients who were not thought to have an infection.

These same researchers then embarked on a second study to see if these unexpected results were valid.[26] In this study, they prospectively removed the spinal implants from fifty consecutive patients with severe pain for unclear reasons following their fusions. These patients had no overt signs of an infection, and again, the presence of bacteria was found in 38 percent of these patients. These researchers knew that this notion of biofilm is not without precedent; other orthopedic procedures, such as failed hip and knee replacements have had similar findings.[27]

In the past few years, there have been additional studies from around the world that have all come to similar conclusions: at least 30 to 40 percent of the spinal implants are infected in those patients with persistent pain post-fusion.[28] So when you take into consideration both systemic and local infection from biofilm, you can now understand that the true infection risk is much higher than the 1 or 2 percent commonly reported. It's also the reason why so many patients continually need opioid pain medication after their fusions. These patients don't want opioids, but the pain is so bad they feel they have no other choice.

The reason the pain is so unbearable is because the body's own immune system is relentlessly attacking the biofilm with inflammatory proteins in the hopes of clearing the local infection. However, the biofilm is often resistant to these attacks, and these inflammatory proteins just continue to build at the interface, creating severe inflammation and chronic pain for patients. It's similar to having a splinter in your finger that you are unable to remove yourself. But imagine that this splinter is the size of a large screw and it's in the middle of your spinal column.

As an educated consumer, if you or a loved one has CLBP and is considering a spinal fusion, you need to weigh the potential risks versus the rewards. In order for you to do so, you need accurate and up-to-date information. Because of these recent findings, many spine surgeons are not only giving antibiotics intravenously at the time of surgery, but also irrigating the surgical site with antibiotics directly in the wound around the implant. The concern with this approach is that no single antibiotic creates a broad-spectrum kill of all microbes and that this practice may fuel the emergence of drug-resistant bacteria called superbugs. So while in the short term, there may be a protective effect, patients may pay for it in the long run.

Given this race to the implant surface together with these new findings that the spine is not a sterile environment, it's not hard to see the potentially disastrous consequences of using implants in spinal surgery. It makes the whole concept of putting any implant into these spaces a risky business, partic-ularly for patients with degenerative disc disease where there may already be a dysbiosis present.

There is a simple scientific explanation of the problem with implants and bacteria. Implants have a high, net-positive surface charge. Bacteria have a high, net-negative surface charge. When you put an implant into the body, the bacteria are unfortunately attracted to it like a magnet (Figure 11). Even with only a few bacteria in the wound, they can attach to the implant, begin to replicate, and start to form biofilm. If this occurs, that implant is essentially rendered useless and can then be a source of chronic pain for patients.

In spinal fusions, biofilm prevents the interface between the implant and the bone from completely assimilating. Instead the body's immune system is constantly trying to fight and knock out the bacterial invasion. This chronic inflammation leads to implant loosening, and then chronic pain which is so frequent after fusions.[29] This loosening is difficult to detect early, so many patients post-fusion are told by their surgeon that their X-rays look fine—"I don't know why you are in so much pain." Now thanks to researchers at HSS like Drs. Cammisa and Abjornson, we are finally beginning to understand that in these patients it's probably related to biofilm formation.

WHY FUSIONS FAIL?

Spinal fusions have such a high failure rate that they've given it a name: Failed Back Surgery Syndrome (FBSS).[30] There are several causes for FBSS:

- Patients developing an acute infection
- Patients developing biofilm formation and the loosening of their spinal implants. Biofilm formation is quickly becoming the number one cause of failed fusions and you need to be aware of this growing problem
- Implants breaking from fatigue or overload
- Nerve damage from inadvertent injury during surgery
- Nerve scarring, commonly referred to as epidural fibrosis
- Herniated discs above or below the fusion from the increase loading of that segment after the fusion
- Poor spinal alignment such as scoliosis or spondylolisthesis
- Narrowing of the spinal canal from stenosis

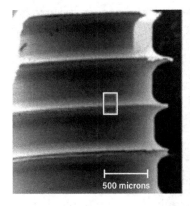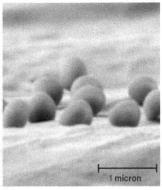

Figure 11: At left is an SEM (Scanning Electron Microscope)
image of a Titanium bone screw at low magnification.
At right is a high magnification SEM image of the region highlighted,
showing the presence of *bacterial* contamination on the implant.
(Courtesy of Orthobond Corporation).

THE INTRADISCAL
MICROBIOME AND PRP

I have been performing intradiscal biologics for over a decade
now, and I have had very few infections, but they can occur.
Anytime you stick a needle in the disc there is a small chance
for an infection. Isabella was a forty-year-old teacher with a
history of CLBP for many years that was refractory to nonsurgical care. She had a somewhat complicated history. She
had a history of cerebral palsy (an injury to the brain that is
a result of decreased blood or oxygen while in the womb).
This left her with leg weakness and spasticity that affected her

gait. Because she spent a great deal of time sitting due to her gait difficulties, she eventually developed a tear in her L5-S1 disc (the lowest disc in your spine). While her MRI did not show any disc herniation or severe degeneration, her pain was severe and disabling.

What complicated her history was that, as a child, she had also developed a condition called hydrocephalus (excess fluid around the brain) that had required a shunt (a plastic tube that runs from the brain to the abdomen) to be placed to reduce the fluid pressure on the brain. While this treated her hydrocephalus, when it was time to remove it they could only safely remove part of the shunt. So she had lived most of her life with this piece of retained plastic tubing in her body.

Isabella's retained shunt is no different than any other implant in the body that could have developed biofilm. Going into the procedure, we knew that this shunt might present a problem, so we took all of the necessary infection precautions and still went ahead with the intradiscal PRP procedure because we thought it would be less risky than spinal surgery.

Unfortunately, within a few weeks of the intradiscal PRP, she developed unremitting back pain, fever, chills, and sweats.

An MRI was obtained which showed signs of an infection in the L5-S1 disc (called spondylodiscitis). A biopsy of the disc was performed and sent to the lab for culture, and the dreaded *C. Acnes* bacteria grew out. She was treated with a sustained course of intravenous antibiotics and thankfully responded, but the disc degenerated, and she was left with persistent back pain. We published this complication to make other physicians aware that infection can occur, even with intradiscal PRP.[31]

In certain spondylodiscitis cases, a spinal fusion is then performed to relieve the pain, but her surgeons were leery because of this retained shunt and their concern for infection. Isabella never had the surgery and lives with persistent back pain. As a physician, you feel terrible when your patient has a complication. It's one of the worst feelings in the world, but rather than give up on a promising procedure, we went back to the lab to study how we can make the intradiscal PRP safer against this *C. Acnes* bacteria. The type of PRP you use really does matter. You will learn more about our research in this area in Chapter 7 Innovating to Improve Outcomes.

In the next chapter, I will explain how regenerative medicine can save your spine—if we can heal your disc, we can end your pain and hopefully avoid spinal surgery.

CHAPTER 6

HOW REGENERATIVE MEDICINE CAN SAVE YOUR SPINE

*"What you do makes a difference, and you have to decide
what kind of difference you want to make."*

—JANE GOODALL

What is *regenerative medicine*? According to the National
Institutes of Health (NIH), it is an emerging area of science
that holds great promise for treating and even curing a variety
of injuries and diseases by using stem cells and other technol-
ogies to repair or replace damaged cells, tissues, and organs.
However, it's not just about stem cells. There are many healing cells and proteins in your body that can stimulate your
natural healing process. There is no drug or surgery that can

come close to mimicking what your body has been already designed to do.

> *With regenerative medicine we take your body's own natural healing powers and put them at the source of the injury to ignite healing—it's that simple.*

Finding the source and understanding the underlying problem is critical for these treatments to be successful. To truly tackle the enormity of the CLBP problem, healthcare systems need a simple solution that can be easily disseminated globally. Regenerative medicine offers not only the hope of a cure for degenerative disc disease, but also a potentially sustainable solution to the most common, most expensive, and most disabling condition we manage as physicians.

It's a complete pivot in thinking on how best to manage the back pain pandemic. In the past, we've thought of herniated discs as "broken" and therefore needing to be cut out. Surgical procedures change the anatomy of your spine permanently. Your back is not broken—your disc has an unhealed wound that needs help to finally heal!

Twelve years ago, my patient James provided me my first glimpse at the profound impact PRP could have on a chronic tendon tear. Watching his Achilles heal completely through two simple PRP injections seemed miraculous. But at the time, the concept of using PRP remained unproven for degenerative disc disease. However, I was buoyed by James's results; tendon tears are also notoriously hard to treat non-surgically, so I continued to investigate. After James, I began to treat my patients with a variety of tendon disorders (rotator cuff, Achilles, patellar tendon, gluteal tendons) with ultrasound-guided PRP injections precisely into the tear. One by one, my patients would improve and be able to return to the sports they loved without any surgery.

By intervening early when the tendon tears were small, we could halt or reverse the tendon from tearing further by creating structural healing.

Conceptually, it wasn't a big leap from there to the notion that this could potentially cure painful tears inside the disc. The same collagen that composes tendons composes the outer rings of the disc—called the annulus fibrosus. But obviously, injecting the inside of a disc carries more risk than a tendon because you're working in the spine.

In medicine when there is a new drug, doctors typically first study it in the lab with what are referred to as preclinical studies. These studies can be both in vitro and in vivo studies.

- In vitro studies are outside a living organism.

- In vivo studies are inside a living organism.

If the researcher builds up enough data to support the premise that the proposed benefits of the drug would outweigh the potential risks, then they can petition the Food and Drug Administration (FDA) to enter into human clinical studies.

> *What's so interesting about regenerative medicine is that it totally disrupts the traditional pharmaceutical model of bringing a new drug to market.*

Because I am using your own cells (referred to as autologous) at point-of-care, on the same day, with what is referred to as "minimal manipulation," these treatments are currently exempt from performing a full FDA trial. That means that these cells cannot be cultured in the lab or boosted with drugs. Clinicians in the US are currently allowed to take your own cells, concentrate them using FDA cleared kits and devices, and put them back into you on the same day. That is why certain types of regenerative treatments are now readily available for patients.

Back in 2010, because of my success with using PRP to treat tendons, I searched worldwide for any data on the use of PRP for degenerative disc disease. There were no clinical studies back then, but there was some compelling preclinical data that begged the question, "Why hasn't anyone tried this yet? It makes so much sense." My excitement about potentially finally finding a solution kept building. The more scientific data I read, the more I felt that this could be the solution I had been searching for for my CLBP patients.

My research team and I went to the literature to see if there was any supportive scientific data for using regenerative medicine to heal your painful disc.

Immediately, we found an interesting study from 2006, where researchers at Rush Medical College in Chicago were the first to show that PRP had a beneficial effect on stimulating cartilage cells.[32] These types of cells, called chondrocytes, are very similar to the cells inside the disc that keep it healthy.

Scientists made PRP from pig's blood and then took their cartilage cells and cultured them in the lab in a broth of PRP where they measured its effects on cell metabolism. These investigators were the first to demonstrate the powerful effects that this "natural cocktail" could have on difficult-to-stimulate cartilage cells. They demonstrated that not only did PRP rev-up the engines of the cells to produce proteins and ignite the healing process, but it did so to a greater degree than cells cultured in blood alone.

These investigators used a commercially available system to make their PRP (similar to what we were using at the time to treat our patients with tendon problems), so nothing too arduous to replicate in the clinical setting. While it was very exciting to see PRP's effects on pig cartilage cells, what about its potential effects on disc cells? We kept searching.

These same researchers also studied the effect of PRP using the same animal model on cells from the disc.[33] Again in an in vitro study culturing cells in the lab, they demonstrated that PRP could even stimulate the cells of the disc to turn on and produce collagen. The effect of the PRP was greater on the cells of the annulus fibrosus (AF) than the nucleus pulposus (NP), but that is exactly what we were searching for. These are the types of cells that would heal the painful tears in the disc. But would it have the same effect on human disc cells?

I then found another study from researchers at Taipei Medical University in Taiwan.[34] They actually studied the effects of **PRP** on human disc cells taken from healthy volunteers. Then researchers cultured these cells in **PRP** and again measured its potential beneficial effects in the lab. Not only were these researchers the first to show the beneficial effects **PRP** could have on human disc cell metabolism, but they also demonstrated that **PRP** could decrease the rate of those cells dying—a process called apoptosis.

> *The more I looked, the more*
> *preclinical data I found to support*
> *my premise of the potential benefits*
> *of injecting PRP inside discs that*
> *were beginning to degenerate.*

These promising studies showed that **PRP** caused beneficial effects on cell proliferation (coming to the wound), increased cell metabolism (producing proteins to repair the wound), and decreased cell death (keeping the disc healthy). In addition, researchers also showed that **PRP** could reduce the number of harmful pro-inflammatory cytokines in the disc, which were responsible for pain and inflammation. This research and research from others gave me enough confidence to proceed to the next step—trying it in actual **CLBP** patients. I felt the risks were low and the potential benefit was significant when compared to undergoing a spinal fusion.

We were now ready to launch a clinical study of intradiscal PRP to treat patients with degenerative disc disease. At the time, I was still heading the Physiatry Department at the Hospital for Special Surgery, so my colleagues and I went to our institutional review board (IRB) to request to study the potential benefits of PRP in the spine. This was a big ask at the time, because there were no prior clinical studies. As a result, none of us really knew the risks. Because of this, I knew that we wanted the most stringent research protocol available, so we chose what is known as a double-blind, randomized controlled trial (DB RCT). I say "we" because research requires a team of health professionals to accomplish a study like this.

Not only is a DB RCT the gold standard in research, it is also the hardest type of study to perform and the most expensive.

Because we were subjecting patients to a new, unproven treatment—and some to no treatment at all—there could be no charge to the patients. As you can imagine, performing these procedures in a hospital setting under anesthesia is an expensive undertaking. Thankfully, I had colleagues willing to donate their time and expertise. But where would I get the necessary resources to fund a study like this? This was a real roadblock to getting the study started.

Again, since this is not a drug study, there was no commercial money to be used to fund it. We had to find another way of funding the study. Just as we began to wonder where we would get the resources, I received a phone call from a grateful patient, Mr. Thomas Kempner, who wanted to have lunch. I didn't ask him; he offered, without any solicitation, $500,000 to support our research in finding a cure for CLBP. I think in life this is called "synchronicity" or maybe something else—"divine intervention." Either way, we now had the resources to begin our DB RCT.

We knew that PRP was not a treatment for every type of CLBP, so we were very strict with who we allowed into the study. We wanted to specifically study patients with early-stage degenerative disc disease who were experiencing severe disabling back pain that had been unresponsive to conservative treatments.

Once selected, we would take them into the procedure room, perform a discogram to confirm that their disc was the source of their pain, and then randomize them into one of two groups: patients who received PRP after the contrast in the discogram and patients who received a placebo (which was just more contrast alone). Neither the patient nor I knew which injection they were receiving—thereby "double-blinding" both the patient and the physician.

Then over an initial period of two months, we tracked their responses with an independent observer who measured: degree of pain relief, functional improvement, and patient satisfaction. In total, we tracked forty-nine patients. For every two patients who received the PRP, one patient was in the control group. This is known as a 2:1 randomization and helped us to enroll patients. We tried a 1:1 randomization schedule but had difficulty getting patients to agree to enroll.

As you can imagine, if you had been in pain for years you would want a better chance to receive a potential beneficial treatment. The other measure we took to increase enrollment was to allow them to cross over into the treatment group. Normally you would like to carry the study out six to twelve months, but again these patients were in severe pain and would not agree to waiting this long to receive a potential life-changing treatment.

So in the crossover-group, if the patient did not see improvement after two months, we unblinded them. If they had received the control and had not improved, we then offered them the intradiscal PRP treatment. Our experience treating tendons has taught us that if you don't see improvement after two months, it's unlikely that it will work. Most patients were willing to wait two months to be unblinded, but three months was pushing it. These nuances are the trials and tribulations of doing a DB RCT, but we got it done and have published our results in a peer-reviewed scientific journal.[35]

The results we saw were powerful. In the first two months, patients who received the PRP were showing significant improvements in pain and function, whereas the control group was not. Further, our patients who had been in the control group and then unblinded also saw significant improvement when they crossed over into the treatment group and received the PRP. There's nothing more convincing than a control subject doing poorly, then receiving the treatment and subsequently thriving. We then followed the treated patients for years, and surprisingly, the majority of patients continued to do well from a single intradiscal injection of their PRP![36] An injection of PRP—their own healing cells and proteins—injected precisely into those painful disc tears ended their pain. These CLBP patients, who on average had pain for four to five years prior to undergoing the procedure, ultimately dropped out of the healthcare system and went back to enjoying their lives. This DB RCT proved intradiscal PRP treatment demonstrated a robust, durable effect, which for a chronic lower back pain treatment has been extremely rare.

We also looked at the MRIs of many of the patients that we treated (Figure 12). It's exceedingly rare in my clinical experience to see these tears, that have lingered for years and failed conservative treatment, resolve on their own. However, in many of the PRP treated patients, the tears improved significantly or disappeared altogether—similar to what we saw with James's Achilles tendon.

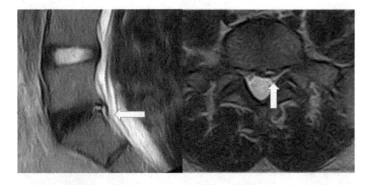

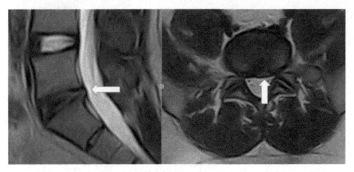

Figure 12: Before (top) and after (bottom) T2-weighted MRI images of one of our patients treated with intradiscal LR-PRP which showed near complete resolution of a chronic tear and disc protrusion within three months. The patient is a professional golfer who had been unable to play his sport and was able to successfully return to full golfing activities.

Interestingly, the pain improvement usually took four to six weeks from the procedure, which is roughly the time it would take for collagen to heal in any area of the body on its own with good blood supply.

I want to point out that these patients were the worst-of-the-worst, having failed multiple trials of conservative care. They had all been in pain for at least four years on average and nothing had worked; their lives were miserable. It was a hard subset of patients to treat, and yet, here we had done just that with a single injection of their own concentrated cells; no drugs, no surgery, *just their own cells.*

Imagine the cost savings at scale that intradiscal PRP can create for healthcare systems.

None of our patients in our study who received the PRP treatment had any adverse reactions such as an infection, progressive disc herniation, or a nerve injury. Either they were no better, or significantly better, but not worse. The patients who did not respond did not burn any treatment bridges by enrolling in the study; they could go on to surgery if they so desired. Out of the forty-nine patients enrolled in the study only six eventually went on to spinal fusion surgery. So we effectively decreased the fusion rate by roughly 80 percent with intradiscal PRP treatment.

Nowadays, if our patients improve partially after an intradiscal PRP injection, they can opt for a booster injection at about the six-month time point. In my clinical experience, this has only further improved our success rates. Unlike steroid injections which can create harmful effects on collagen, these regenerative treatments can have a cumulative positive effect on tissue regeneration with repeat injections. Our research goal is to find ways to optimize the intradiscal PRP treatment to be one and done with a greater than 90 percent success rate.

As we have learned, the disc is a difficult structure to heal. Until we come up with more powerful regenerative treatments, sometimes the simplest step is just to repeat the procedure another time with PRP. This has to be weighed against the risks of another injection into the disc, so it is rare that we would do this more than twice in the same patient. By far the majority of our patients respond to only one treatment.

Intradiscal PRP has become our main treatment for patients with degenerative disc disease at RSI.

Take Harvey's case for example: he came to me for a consultation about what to do for his CLBP after suffering for six years. At this point, Harvey was in such severe pain that it was challenging for him to even sit, and he carried a cushion wherever he went. Throughout those six years of disabling pain, Harvey had tried every conservative avenue: seven

MRIs, multiple trials of oral medications, more than fifty physical therapy sessions, and nineteen spinal injection procedures (mostly epidural steroids).

Imagine—after all of that, nothing had given him any significant pain relief; he was miserable, and his life was falling apart! As a prominent trial attorney, he found that he could no longer even concentrate on his work. A spinal fusion seemed like the only option left for him. That's the moment we met. Harvey was referred to me by another patient of mine.

When I looked at the MRI of his spine, he clearly had a significant problem with two of the lower discs. They were torn, protruding, and beginning to degenerate—a classic degenerative cascade. So we discussed intradiscal PRP as an option to consider before the spinal fusion. What did he have to lose? If it didn't work, he could always still get the fusion. Harvey agreed.

So we injected his two degenerative discs with PRP, and within six weeks his life was changed. Not only did his pain diminish significantly, but now he was able to get back to exercising and concentrating at work. He was able to return to most of the activities that CLBP had robbed from him for the past six years. It has been over three years since his procedure, and he continues to do very well with nothing more than some ongoing exercises.

Now enjoying life, Harvey sent me his thirty-year-old son, Michael, who lived in California. Michael had developed similar, disabling chronic lower back pain. Luckily, his loving dad stepped right in and flew him out to see us. He did not want his son to endure the same saga that he'd gone through. I performed the same regenerative procedure his father had just had, and Michael too improved significantly. Michael's experience, however, was completely different in significant ways: he had not had seven MRIs—just one; he had not had nineteen spinal injections—just one; and he had not had numerous physical therapy sessions or numerous trials of oral medications. It's been over three years now, and Michael is also doing extremely well.

Think of the years of potential disability Michael escaped. Think of the potential risk he avoided because he did not have multiple, unnecessary procedures. Although small, each spinal procedure carries some risk for bleeding, infection, and/ or nerve injury. These risks always have to be weighed with the patient before any procedure, including these regenerative treatments. Additionally, think of the significant cost savings by hitting the bullseye early on in his disease process. This is the power of regenerative medicine, and it's why I am so excited to share this information with you. We finally have a treatment approach to CLBP that makes sense and puts the patient's needs above all others.

Since our initial DB RCT study in 2016, it has been encouraging to witness other investigators from around the world publishing similar encouraging results.[37] [38] [39] Akeda et al recently published another DB RCT comparing intradiscal platelet releasate to intradiscal corticosteroid injections in patients with degenerative disc disease. Platelet releasate is slightly different from the type of PRP we used in our study. It does not contain white blood cells or fibrin (which is the natural glue in your blood) but it does contain the growth factors inside the platelets.

While there are several limitations to this study (no control group, only sixteen patients, corticosteroid injected with 2 ml saline, not a leukocyte-rich PRP (LR-PRP), and no statistical difference in outcome), they found that over a sixty week period the PRP group did experience a greater degree of pain relief and functional improvement. This makes intradiscal PRP the only orthobiologic treatment option with two supportive RCT studies.

There was, however, a very recent single-blind randomized controlled study of intradiscal PRP that did not show a significant difference between the treatment group and the control group.[40] Both the PRP and the control groups showed modest improvement in pain and function after intradiscal injection. These authors therefore concluded that intradiscal PRP was of no benefit.

If we take a deeper dive into this study, there were some serious flaws in their methodology that I believe confounded their conclusion that intradiscal PRP was no better than their control: they used a leukocyte poor PRP, they injected only a small amount (1 cc) of a low platelet concentration PRP, they did not quantify what they injected, they did not use contrast to demonstrate flow into the annular tears, they used saline and antibiotics as the control, and they excluded a very important subset of patients (Modic 1 changes) from their study.

In our experience, it is exactly this subset of patients (MC1) that has responded the best to intradiscal LR-PRP. In addition, using saline and antibiotics really are not a negative control as you will learn. These agents have an antibacterial effect that may have improved some of the patients in the control group thereby confounding their results. The type of

PRP used to treat degenerative disc disease really does matter. There continues to be a need for more rigorous research on intradiscal PRP for patients with degenerative disc disease.

It is rare to achieve such good results with a first-out-of-box PRP therapy like we used in our initial study. We are continuing to research and innovate better ways of delivering the PRP inside the disc, as well as better ways to concentrate the platelets to even higher levels and improve outcomes further. You will learn more about the advancements we have made to further improve our intradiscal PRP success rates in the next chapter.

> *Remember Beth? Imagine what her life would have been like if these regenerative treatments had been available at the time she needed them.*

You, however, do not have to wait. I, along with other like-minded physicians, have been performing and perfecting these exciting intradiscal PRP injections for the past twelve years now. This is not something new or theoretical; we have now treated over one thousand CLBP patients with a special kind of PRP especially designed for the disc to kill two birds with one stone, offering CLBP patients new hope to end their pain.

In the next chapter you will learn:

- How we have collaborated with industry experts to develop a PRP system that can produce higher concentrations of platelets than the leading PRP systems on the market

- How we have also invented a curved intradiscal catheter that can precisely place this higher concentration PRP into the areas of the disc where the tears reside (the annulus fibrosus) better than the standard technique

- How the combination of these two advancements is optimizing our clinical outcomes so that more patients can benefit to a greater degree

CHAPTER 7

INNOVATING TO IMPROVE CLINICAL OUTCOMES

"Failure is success in progress"

—**ALBERT EINSTEIN,** 1879–1955

Overall, while the results we were achieving with intradiscal PRP were unlike any other CLBP treatment in the past, there were still a fair number of patients that did not improve— roughly 40 percent. This was not good enough, so my team and I went back to the drawing board. How could we optimize our PRP preparation and delivery to improve the odds for success?

Innovating is an iterative process—you learn as much from your failures as you do from your successes.

In our initial double-blinded randomized controlled study (DB RCT) of intradiscal PRP at HSS, we concentrated the platelets in our PRP preparation to approximately three to five times the normal baseline concentration—meaning if your baseline platelet concentration was about two hundred thousand platelets, we were achieving concentrations in the PRP between six hundred thousand to one million per microliter. When we perform intradiscal PRP, we use a total volume of about two milliliters—so we are injecting billions of your platelets into each disc to ignite the healing cascade!

The simplest next step was to increase that concentration of platelets further. By now there were more and more companies producing PRP kits that could concentrate well beyond those initial levels of the first PRP kits we used. It seemed logical that more platelets would translate into a higher delivery of healing growth factors, but we needed to test that hypothesis: could patients with more severe disc disease just require a greater degree of growth factors to obtain pain relief? Other researchers using in vivo animal studies suggested that higher concentrations of platelets might even translate into regeneration.[41]

One of the confusions within the field of regenerative medicine is the variability in the PRP product.

Each patient has not only a unique platelet count but also a unique growth factor composition inside their platelets. There are also many different methods available to prepare PRP: from different spin protocols for centrifugation to over fifty different commercially cleared PRP systems, all producing a varied PRP end product. In order to optimize our clinical outcomes, we first needed to focus on reducing this variability and quantify what we were actually injecting.

When we opened RSI, one of the first pieces of equipment we bought was a hemocytometer. A hemocytometer is a machine that can actually do a blood count of cells at the bedside. This enabled us to count the patient's baseline platelet count, process their PRP, and then take a small sample of the PRP and retest their platelet count so we would know exactly what we were injecting. Not only does this machine test platelet counts, but it also counts white blood cells and other types of cells in the blood. This enables us to not only measure the dose of cells in the PRP but also the ratio over baseline that we were able to achieve with that particular PRP system on every patient. Now, we have the ability to quantify our dose of platelets and other cells in the PRP we inject to see if it correlates with outcome. This effectively allowed us to measure the "dose" of platelets we were injecting, similar to a drug discovery program. This is part of the quality-control program we have in place at RSI.

With our new quality-control system, we found that with certain newer PRP systems we could achieve platelet concentrations of greater than ten times the patient's baseline—sometimes even higher—on a consistent basis simply by lowering the volume of plasma (the protein portion of the blood). It's actually very simple to do and easy to translate for others, which facilitates widespread dissemination.[42]

Now we were ready to put this new higher-concentration (essentially double the concentration) PRP to the test. We performed what is referred to as a retrospective registry study.

We looked back at the number of patients we had treated over the past few years with this higher concentration PRP and found about forty-five patients who were over a year out. We were able to get data on thirty-seven of those patients, which is an acceptable follow-up rate of over 80 percent.

Then, we compared their results—pain relief, functional improvement, and patient satisfaction—to our historic DB

RCT results to see if they were equal, worse, or potentially better.

> *Not only did we see greater degrees of*
> *pain relief and functional improvement,*
> *but our patient satisfaction rates*
> *were now over 80 percent.*[43]

The results were even more encouraging than our first study. The simple step of doubling the concentration of platelets in the PRP improved our outcomes by over 20 percent!

Unfortunately, one of the patients in the study, Isabella, had a complication of a spinal infection. As you recall, she was infected with the same bacteria that you have already learned about—*C. Acnes.* In our attempt to concentrate the platelets to higher levels, some patients received a leukocyte-poor PRP, and this is the type of PRP she received.

Isabella's case prompted us to go even further in our research to see what type of PRP is the safest. We believe it matters a great deal for reasons I am about to explain.

ARE WE KILLING TWO BIRDS
WITH ONE STONE?

"First, do no harm" is something we physicians are taught in medical school, but the reality in practice is that every treatment is a double-edged sword. Any treatment, even something as safe as using your own cells, has the potential to do harm.

As I mentioned earlier, the disc is an unforgiving space. All we can do is mitigate the risk to the best of our abilities for patients. Any time you put a needle anywhere, there is a small risk of developing an infection. We wanted to see what more we could do to reduce the risk so that the potential benefits of this promising new procedure would significantly outweigh the potential risks.

We already knew, from the literature and our own personal experience, that *C. Acnes* was the culprit in many of the infections associated with intradiscal biologic procedures.[44] So we went back to the lab and cultured the *C. Acnes* bacteria in different types of PRP—**leukocyte-rich** (**LR-PRP**) versus **leukocyte-poor** (**LP-PRP**).

We cultured the *C. Acnes* bacteria for up to forty-eight hours and found that the LR-PRP did indeed create greater kill rates than the LP-PRP.[45] Now we have more evidence for what we believe to be not only the most effective type of PRP for degenerative disc disease, but also the safest. Our clinical experience reflects this safety finding.

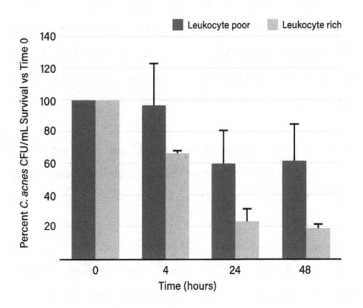

Figure 13: Is a graph representing the effect of a leukocyte poor vs leukocyte rich PRP on the growth of bacteria (*C. Acnes*) in culture over time. Our study showed a greater suppression of bacterial growth with a leukocyte-rich PRP.

It is my belief that we may actually be killing two birds with one stone with our intradiscal LR-PRP. Not only are we igniting the body's natural healing response in the disc, but the high levels of white blood cells in the LR-PRP could also be suppressing the overgrowth of certain types of bacteria associated with causing the disc to be painful and degenerate —*C. Acnes.*

Stacey was a thirty-two-year-old woman who presented to my office with severe CLBP that had not responded to traditional treatments. What was unusual about her history was that she couldn't attribute the onset of her pain to any specific event.

She rated the pain as an eight out of ten. She had a two-year-old daughter that she was having a difficult time caring for because she couldn't lift her. So we obtained an MRI of her lumbar spine to see what was going on. It revealed two degenerative discs with significant inflammatory response in the vertebral bodies (called Modic 1 changes). Modic changes are believed to represent inflammatory changes in the vertebral body from degenerative discs that may have a chronic local infection.

She had already failed oral medications, chiropractic care, acupuncture, and an epidural steroid injection which gave only short-term pain relief. Spinal surgery, she said, was a last resort. So we discussed the pros and cons of intradiscal LR-PRP in her case, and she agreed to the procedure.

Collaborating with industry partners (Andy McGillicuddy from Cervos Medical and Barry Zimble from Ranfac Corporation), we have been able to invent a new PRP system that we believe will improve outcomes of intradiscal PRP. We wanted a PRP system that could concentrate not only the platelets but also the bacteria-fighting white blood cells to higher levels than previous systems. This type of collaboration, as you will learn more about in the next chapter, will help us shift the treatment paradigm towards regenerative medicine.

To give you an idea of the potency of the PRP, we injected well over five billion platelets and one hundred million white blood cells (WBCs) into each of her discs. Think about the thousands of healing proteins in the platelets and the anti-bacterial power of the WBCs exactly where they are needed. Finally, we have a treatment for the root cause plaguing so many patients with degenerative disc disease. This is what regenerative medicine is all about.

At first, Stacey's pain was worse from the pressure of the injection into a painful structure and the inflammatory response these cells cause in the first few days, but within weeks she started to improve. When we repeated the MRI three months later, not only was the majority of her pain gone, so were those Modic 1 changes (Figure 14).

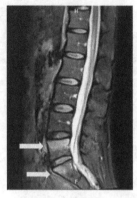
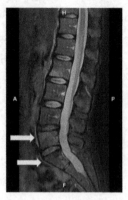

SIGNIFICANT
IMPROVEMENT
IN MC1 CHANGES
AND CLINICAL
SYMPTOMS AFTER
INTRADISCAL
LR-PRP L4-5 &
L5-S1

Figure 14: Before (left) and after (right) T2-weighted MRI images
of Stacey's lumbar spine treated with intradiscal LR-PRP which showed
near complete resolution of the Modic 1 changes (bright signal
in the bone represented by the arrows which resolved).

We have treated so many patients now just like Stacey. I do believe we are killing two birds with one stone, which is why intradiscal injection of a LR-PRP is offering new hope to patients suffering from CLBP.

Now that we've identified what we believe to be the safest, most effective intradiscal biologic—how else can we potentially improve patient outcomes?

PRECISION CELL DELIVERY

One of the things I have learned over the past three decades of performing interventional spinal procedures is that you need to deliver the therapeutic agent as close to the problem as possible to create the greatest benefit. Even with an epidural steroid injection, the best effects are when it is placed precisely between the inflamed disc and nerve root.

The problem when we perform an intradiscal injection is that we are placing a straight needle into a round structure. The most painful tears inside the disc are in the back portion of the disc. As a result, we are often unable to get a straight needle into that area consistently. Most of the time the needle is placed in the middle of the disc and, when we inject, we hope that the LR-PRP fills the tears. The problem with this approach is not all annular tears communicate with the center of the disc. So there are significant limitations in using just a straight-needle technique for delivering LR-PRP inside the disc.

Hope is not a strategy we like in medicine.

We prefer to have a reliable means of precisely placing the cells as closely into the tears as possible. So again we collaborated with Andy, Barry, and one of Ranfac's engineers, Cameron, to develop the first intradiscal catheter capable of precisely delivering biologics directly into the posterior annulus fibrosus, where most painful tears occur.

Anthony is a sixty-three-year-old patient of mine that I had been seeing for over eight years for his CLBP. His pain wasn't always severe—it waxed and waned depending upon the amount of activity he did. He didn't recall any inciting event. The more he worked out, skied, or sat, the worse his pain became. It was also associated with leg pain and numbness down his right leg which was very concerning to him.

His MRI eight years ago showed a right-sided annular tear and disc protrusion at the L4-5 level. While he responded to epidural steroid injections and physical therapy, the pain would gradually come back after a few months. When I recently saw him back in follow-up for the same symptoms, the MRI showed exactly the same tear in the same disc. So, I discussed with him the option of intradiscal LR-PRP precisely delivered with our new curved intradiscal catheter.

He was willing, and within three months after the procedure, not only did his symptoms of eight years resolve, but the annular tear healed on his follow-up MRI (Figure 15).

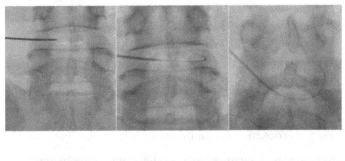

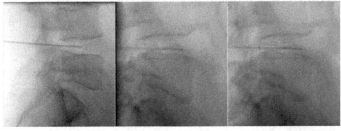

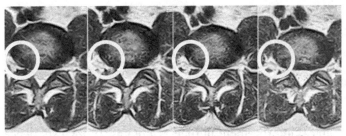

| Chronic untreated tear for 8 years | 1 month post healing | 2 months post healing | 3 months post healing |

Figure 15: Anthony's intradiscal procedure using a curved catheter (top fluoroscopic images) to place the LR-PRP as close to the disc tear as possible. We followed his recovery with monthly MRIs which showed healing of the annular tear (circle) over a three month period.

A PROMISING FUTURE

If you are reading this book for yourself, a friend, or a loved one who is suffering from CLBP, it's important to know about intradiscal LR-PRP. It is the first treatment that targets two potential root causes; painful unhealed annular tears and the overgrowth of harmful bacteria that contributes to degenerative disc disease. Hopefully, as we gain a better understanding of how to optimize these regenerative therapies, we can use them not just to repair but to regenerate discs. Treatments that just relieve pain and do not create healing structural changes are only palliative, not curative. By really harnessing the innate regenerative capacity of your body, for your benefit, you will hopefully be able to live a life free of back pain. That is the "holy grail" of spinecare!

We are continually seeing patients we have treated with positive structural changes after intradiscal LR-PRP, not just clinical improvement in their symptoms. In my experience, there seems to be a linear relationship with the degree of healing and the degree of pain improvement. In other words, if the tear in the disc is 50 percent healed the patient is 50 percent better; if it is 100 percent healed they are 100 percent better.

This information is invaluable because a treatment that makes a structural change in the disc is a potential cure.

We never thought the disc could heal on its own, but now we know that that common belief in the medical establishment is not true. The injured disc just needs the precise delivery of healing cells and proteins, just like any other structure in the body. Your body is your best surgeon!

One of the questions I hear from patients is whether or not my aged-degenerated disc is capable of healing. It's an excellent question that was recently answered by researchers from Berlin, Germany.[46] At the time of surgery, they harvested annulus fibrosus cells (AFCs) from discs that showed early and late signs of degeneration and compared their response to PRP in the lab. What these investigators were able to demonstrate was that even AFCs from degenerated discs retained their regenerative capacity to proliferate, migrate, and produce collagen.

I believe, after seeing many patients like Anthony over the past decade, that a paradigm shift will occur in how we manage CLBP, a shift towards regenerative medicine.

If you have been struggling with CLBP you do not need to wait. These intradiscal LR-PRP treatments are readily available for you now. We have made this complete paradigm shift at RSI. But how do we create this shift on a larger level so that more patients can benefit from this discovery?

At first, I was a skeptic that this treatment would even work. That is why I have waited for over a decade to perform the necessary research to evaluate its efficacy and safety. I finally feel confident spreading the word about intradiscal LR-PRP, but as you can imagine, there are many naysayers and entrenched players that will resist this paradigm shift away from drugs and surgery toward regenerative medicine.

The path of any new medical treatment has historically been fraught with many landmines to navigate. Innovating to improve outcomes is an iterative process that requires collaboration. I believe we have finally found the secret recipe to treat CLBP on a global basis: high concentration LR-PRP precisely delivered inside the disc with an intradiscal curved catheter. In the next chapter, you will learn not only how best we can navigate these barriers to change in the medical community, but also how we can use a process called vertical collaboration to shift the treatment paradigm towards regenerative medicine.

CHAPTER 8

COLLABORATING TO OVERCOME BARRIERS TO CHANGE

"Intelligence is the ability to adapt to change."

—**STEPHEN HAWKING**, 1942–2018

The nineteenth century philosopher Arthur Schopenhauer said that all truths have to pass through three stages: the first one being **ridicule**, the second one being **violent opposition**, and the third one is that it is accepted as being **self-evident**. The medical community can historically be tough on physicians who are bringing out new ideas and theories on medical conditions. I think intradiscal LR-PRP is unfortunately in the first stage, but that doesn't have to affect your healthcare decision. This treatment is readily available now, and if I was experiencing CLBP it's what I would pursue before considering any spinal surgery.

Let's back up for a moment and look at a brief history of how the treatment of ulcers, for example, has evolved over time. Up until 1982, doctors believed that peptic ulcers were caused by spicy foods and stress. Around this time, Dr. J. Robins Warren observed that a bacterium was present in about 50 percent of his patients who had their stomachs biopsied[47]. He joined forces with Dr. Barry J. Marshall, and together they initiated a study where they biopsied the stomachs of one hundred patients who were thought to have ulcers.

They discovered a previously unknown bacterium called *Helicobacter pylori (H. pylori)* and found that it was almost always present in patients suffering from peptic ulcers. They began to question the notion that stress and spicy foods were the culprits doctors believed them to be at the time. They proposed that it was actually a bacterial overgrowth of the stomach, dysbiosis inside the stomach.

Even with their clear scientific evidence, the medical community was so entrenched in the idea that lifestyle was the cause, that their findings initially did not amount to a shift in treatment protocols; no one adopted this new mode of thinking. In fact, they were ridiculed and violently opposed by some of their colleagues. The medical community was under the belief that the stomach, due to its acidity, was a sterile environment.

So what did these physicians do? They persisted, and to prove their point, Dr. Marshall deliberately infected himself with the bacterium, and sure enough he developed a peptic ulcer.

Today, it has become widely accepted (self-evident) that *H. pylori* is not just a major cause of ulcers but is also a major risk factor for developing gastric cancer.[48] This discovery has created a paradigm shift in the treatment of ulcers. Instead of relying on surgery and the chronic use of antacids, the "cure" has become antibiotics to reduce the bacterial overgrowth and actually heal the ulcer. These dedicated physicians, after being initially ridiculed by the medical establishment for years, were later recognized and awarded the Nobel Prize for their prescient discovery in 2005.[49]

FINANCIAL BARRIERS

After discovering through our research the dramatic impact of these promising regenerative treatments, I was anxious to bring its healing powers to my patients at large. Easier said than done.

First, the financial barriers to bringing treatments to patients were immediately evident. Insurance companies consider most regenerative treatments "experimental," and as such, refuse to cover the procedure. Because of the expense, performing these procedures in a hospital setting was not going to work. The out-of-pocket expenses for patients to just walk into a hospital surgical suite and recovery room are prohibitive.

I had to come up with a more cost-effective solution. So I made the leap to venture out on my own and create an independent private clinic where I could safely perform these procedures at a reduced cost compared to the hospital. RSI was built specifically to study regenerative orthopedic treatments to heal ailing spines and joints.

There were many uncertainties about this transition away from the security of a large hospital. At RSI we could now offer these promising regenerative treatments at significantly less cost than at the hospital. RSI was built with the concept of how we would want to be treated if we were the patient. We wanted to eliminate some of the pain points for patients: long wait times for appointments, multiple days off from work to obtain diagnostic tests or treatments, and an impersonal environment.

At RSI all our diagnostic imaging needs and procedure suites are on site—so our patients can be evaluated, receive their imaging studies, and often receive their treatments in just one visit. Same-day diagnosis and same-day treatment. It's a very efficient system of musculoskeletal care that respects our patients' needs and time. Having our own MRI on-site has enabled us to see firsthand the structural healing effects these treatments have on the spines, joints, and tendons we treat with regenerative medicine.

While we have already made this paradigm shift toward regenerative medicine at RSI, it is going to take a lot more than just one site in NYC to make that shift a reality. Thankfully, I have witnessed successful paradigm shifts in other areas of life—again from a world outside of medicine, the regenerative farming movement.

LESSONS LEARNED FROM A FARMER

My wife, Paula, has an interest in organic farming and about seven years ago invited me to attend the Northeast Organic Farmer Association's (NOFA) annual conference. I just went to keep her company, not knowing what was going to happen next. The very first lecture when we walked through the doors was from their keynote speaker, a farmer named John Ickerd. John is also a professor emeritus of agricultural economics at the University of Missouri, and he has authored two books: *Sustainable Capitalism, A Return to Common Sense*; and *Small Farms are Real Farms*.

John has been farming his entire seventy-five years in one way or another. He grew up on a small dairy farm in the Midwest at a time when farming communities were collaborative, small, and personal. John also spent a large portion of his professional career teaching at the university level about the importance of feeding the world through the corporatization of farming.

When he got up to speak, he opened by describing how he was born on a small dairy farm, spent most of his life in farming, and then taught farming at the University level. He then said, "I thought I knew what was best, but I GOT IT ALL WRONG." That opening definitely got my attention.

He went on to tell the audience how he had spent the majority of his professional career teaching about the importance of creating a mass food source to try to fight world hunger, and how the large farming corporations with greater resources were better equipped than small farms to accomplish this. He then began to share how this change from small farms to large farms owned by corporations definitely increased food production but came at a significant cost.

These large farming corporations employed farming tactics that extracted and exploited not only the land, but also the small farms that used to farm them. They destroyed many of these small farming communities that were the backbone of our country. They introduced the use of pesticides and farming practices that have threatened the safety of the food we all eat and created significant health risks for all of us. In the drive to increase volume and profits, food safety, value, and sustainability were lost.

I edged forward in my seat as I began to listen more intently. I was beginning to see the similarities between what happened to farming and what has been happening to healthcare in this country. This is particularly evident in how we have mismanaged lower back pain with over-medicating and over-surgerizing patients—this so-called corporatization of back pain. If you are interested in learning more, read *Crooked: Outwitting the Back Pain Industry and Getting On the Road to Recovery* by Cathryn Jakobson Ramin, an investigative journalist. Read the chapter on *The Opioid Wars*, a great example of how corporate greed ruined many patients' lives.

Ickerd argued that these large farming corporations had very little capacity to make social and ethical decisions for the greater good. These corporations were not necessarily evil, but certainly did not make ethics their priority. Economics is what primarily drove their decisions. Rather than keep the small farming communities intact and collaborate with them, they just bought up farms and extracted and exploited what they could from them, leaving many of these farming communities in the wake.

To extract and exploit has and always will be simpler in the short-term than making long-term investments in sustainability and collaboration. Too big becomes too impersonal. Professor Ickerd would go on to say, "For farming to be sustainable it has to be regenerative and personal." OK now he really got my attention, because this is exactly what I believe we need to do to improve musculoskeletal healthcare in this country.

The similarities to what has happened to our healthcare system here in the US are concerning. Private physician practices used to be the norm and were the backbone of healthcare;

they were the foundation of the doctor-patient relationship. Physicians were integral members of keeping their communities healthy. It was a very personal relationship. I knew this firsthand because I grew up in a family of physicians. My dad was a doctor in private practice, and my mom was a nurse. All four kids became physicians. We grew up in medicine and were exposed to some of the best, most ethical physicians at our own dinner table. They would preach to us about the need to protect the sanctity of the doctor-patient relationship.

However, over the past decade there has been a dangerous trend in healthcare that does not bode well for patients: the corporatization of physician practices. According to the *Physicians Foundation Survey,* the number of physicians self-identifying as independent private practices has decreased to just 32 percent in 2016. Similarly, the number identifying as being employees of either a hospital or large medical group has increased to 57 percent. This trend is only escalating because of the pandemic effect and is in contrast to the late 1980s when over 70 percent were private practice physicians.

I had come to the NOFA conference mainly with no expectations. I left feeling inspired by Ickerd's words because every time he used the word farming, I could have substituted the word healthcare. We have a social and ethical imperative to create a sustainable solution for patients with CLBP. For this healthcare solution to occur it has to be "regenerative and personal," just like Ickerd said.

The similarities between what Ickerd was preaching regarding farming resonated with my feelings about my own practice. In fact, those feelings are in great part what prompted me to open RSI. RSI is a good start, but it is not enough to create a paradigm shift. So how do we move the needle further? It is through a system called vertical collaboration.

A SPINECARE PARADIGM SHIFT THROUGH VERTICAL COLLABORATION

Vertical collaboration is a business strategy in which two or more organizations from different levels or stages in the supply chain share their responsibilities, resources, and performance information to serve relatively similar end customers; in this case the end customer is the patient with CLBP. In order for the shift to occur, the needs of the patient have to come first, and that philosophy has to be shared by all involved in providing healthcare: the physicians, allied health professionals, hospitals, industry, and insurance companies.

The patient is at the top of this vertical system of collaboration with the physician. There is no more important collaborative relationship than the doctor-patient relationship. This is where it all starts, and the other players have to support, protect, and respect this relationship for optimal healthcare to occur. The corporatization of healthcare is threatening the foundation of the doctor-patient relationship.

Currently, our healthcare system is more about vertical competition rather than collaboration. There are many entities competing for that patient with CLBP, and not all of them have the patient's best interest at heart.

Pharmaceutical companies touting their drugs as the answer, medical device companies wanting to increase the sales of their spinal fusion implants, hospitals relying too heavily on surgical revenues to survive, and the nefarious characters pushing "stem cell" treatments from amniotic products without any supportive data to back up their claims—all stand to benefit from perpetuating this cycle. What's a patient with CLBP to do? Who do they turn to for advice? They turn to a physician with whom they have developed a personal and trusting relationship. This is where vertical collaboration begins and ends.

Once a trusting doctor-patient relationship is established, there then has to be collaboration among all of the other players to help that patient get better. It's that simple. Anything that threatens the doctor-patient relationship has to be either eliminated or modified. Knowledge has to be shared freely between healthcare providers without any strings attached. Clinical outcome data has to be analyzed independently without commercial bias. Industry has to make products that are safe and effective, even if it costs more to do so. For a healthcare system to be honorable and sustainable, the needs of the patient have to always come first.

VERTICAL COLLABORATION: A PATIENT FIRST APPROACH

Remember my very first intradiscal PRP patient, Jeff? He struggled to find effective care for his CLBP, a story you might relate to, but ultimately benefited as a direct result of vertical collaboration that put the patient's needs first.

By the time I saw him, Jeff had suffered with back pain for over two years and tried all the available conservative treatment options. He told me about the struggle he had trying to decide if he should go ahead with a spinal fusion. I was his last hope. Neither one of us knew if intradiscal PRP would be of any benefit, but we decided to collaborate on his treatment trial. He benefited from being collaborative in trying a new treatment and ultimately never needed that spinal fusion.

The power of regenerative medicine is real, and we are in the early stages of a paradigm shift in how we can better manage this global condition. It's going to take time, but this shift is already beginning to happen. It's beginning because patients with CLBP are seeking better and safer treatment alternatives and are willing to collaborate with innovative, like-minded physicians. Be curious as a patient and trust your intuition as you decide on what is best for you.

We do not yet know for sure if our regenerative treatments halt the progression of degeneration, but it is my belief, based on the patients we have treated, that it certainly has the potential. Time will tell. Wouldn't it be remarkable if these treatments not only provide substantial pain relief but also halt or even reverse disc degeneration? This is why I am so excited to share this information with you about how regenerative medicine can save your spine and change the treatment paradigm for CLBP.

However, for this paradigm shift to really gain more momentum, it is going to be so important for physicians to collaborate not only with the patient, but also with each other, with researchers, with the FDA, hospitals, insurance payers, politicians, and industry to better improve the safety and clinical outcomes of these regenerative procedures. These procedures need to be democratized so that anyone suffering from CLBP can have this treatment option before crossing the Rubicon into the surgical maze.

My prediction is that regenerative medicine is going to change how we manage patients with CLBP in the years to come for the better. Think about the millions of lives improved and the billions of healthcare dollars saved when a simple outpatient injection of your own LR-PRP replaces many of those costly hospital-based spinal surgeries. Spinal surgery will still be necessary for some patients, but there will not be nearly as many surgeries as are done currently. Think about how LR-PRP kills two birds with one stone, finally offering patients a safe opioid-sparing treatment option that is readily available today.

Regenerative medicine and regenerative farming have more in common than we realized. We can learn a lot from people like John Ickerd and the small farmers involved in the organic farming movement. The only way we are going to create a meaningful, sustainable change in how we manage this vexatious problem will be through a healthcare system of vertical collaboration, not competition. If your healthcare provider is not being collaborative, find one that is. In the next chapter you will learn how best to do that.

CHAPTER 9

HOW TO FIND A REGENERATIVE SPINE SPECIALIST

"Only those who regard healing as the ultimate goal of their efforts can, therefore, be designated as physicians."

—DR. RUDOLPH VIRCHOW, 1821–1902

Now that you have learned about this new intradiscal LR-PRP treatment option, what do you do with this information? How do you find a regenerative spine specialist that can help you be evaluated for this treatment? Most people, let alone many physicians, do not even know about this treatment option yet. It was my intention to share with you as much knowledge as I can to help you make an informed decision. Remember, you always have a choice when it comes to your healthcare.

If you are frustrated with the lack of improvement you have had with traditional treatments, then it is time to turn toward exploring your regenerative medicine options.

I will help you navigate this somewhat complicated system, but first you need to decide that this is what you want. Once you have decided to proceed, I can provide you with the necessary steps to get the care you deserve. The next critical step is choosing the right provider. The healthcare provider you choose to see first can make an enormous difference in your ultimate outcome.

Remember Jennifer from Chapter One? Jennifer was first referred to a rheumatologist. The rheumatologist by nature is going to focus on the autoimmune aspect because that's what they are trained to do. But Jennifer did not meet all of the criteria for the diagnosis she received of ankylosing spondylitis but nevertheless was treated for over a year with powerful immunosuppressant drugs with no benefit. Her physicians discounted or didn't even notice the tear in her L5-S1 disc, which ended up being the cause of all of her pain.

So how do you find a "regenerative spine specialist"? Since there are not yet any accredited programs specifically in regenerative medicine, you are going to have to do some detective work. There is an emerging field of medicine called interventional orthobiologics. It is a group of like-minded physicians from various medical specialties (PM&R, orthopedics, radiology, anesthesiology, neurology, internal medicine, and family practice) that have achieved additional training in image-guided minimally invasive musculoskeletal procedures employing your own cells.

I see a similar shift occurring in spinecare to what has occurred in cardiology: a shift away from open surgeries to minimally invasive interventional orthobiologic procedures. What has happened in the field of interventional cardiology is unbelievable. Open heart surgeries have been largely replaced by these minimally invasive image-guided interventional cardiology procedures. You can even now replace each heart valve percutaneously!

At RSI all of our physicians are board certified, fellowship-trained interventional physiatrists.

WHAT'S AN INTERVENTIONAL PHYSIATRIST?

Interventional physiatrists are medical doctors who have not only completed an accredited medical school and residency program in Physical Medicine & Rehabilitation (PM&R), but also additional fellowship training in interventional orthopedic procedures. So not only do they possess the necessary skills to perform a detailed musculoskeletal history and physician exam and review appropriate musculoskeletal imaging studies, but they also can perform these interventional orthopedic procedures. Similar to an interventional cardiologist delivering stents to a clogged blood vessel in your heart, these interventional physiatrists are performing similar procedures in spines and joints.

Historically, many of these interventional spinal procedures were for delivering contrast dye, anesthetics, and anti-inflammatory medications; but it's now shifting more towards regenerative treatments. Physiatrists have broad training in neuromusculoskeletal conditions. At one extreme, they are trained to care for patients with spinal cord injuries, and at the other, they are trained to manage patients with CLBP.

Physiatrists are trained to not only diagnose the specific causes of your CLBP but can also make sure you are optimizing all reasonable non-surgical treatment options before considering any surgery. Physiatrists are rehabilitation experts and will work closely with your physical therapist to ensure your exercise program post-procedure is personalized for your full recovery. What's particularly appealing about an interventional physiatrist is that they can manage your whole spinecare from start to finish.

HOW TO CONDUCT AN
ONLINE SEARCH FOR PROVIDERS

How do you separate out the physicians who are truly capable of performing intradiscal LR-PRP?

There are also a number of physician organizations that I recommend which maintain a list of physicians that could be offering these procedures in your area: the American Academy of Physical Medicine & Rehabilitation (AAPM&R) website (*https://www.aapmr.org/*), Interventional Orthobiologics Foundation (*https://interventionalorthobiologics.org/*), and the Spinal Intervention Society (*https://www.spineintervention.org*).

Preferably you want to seek a regenerative spine specialist who has been performing these intradiscal PRP procedures for at least three to five years. Don't be afraid to ask the following questions:

- What types of cells are you actually injecting into my spine?

- Are you using intradiscal PRP?

- Are you using a leukocyte-rich PRP?

- How are you preparing your PRP?

- What quality control systems do you have in place?

- Are you using FDA approved PRP kits?

- Are you quantifying the number of cells you are injecting?

- Are you including any antibiotics to prevent the risk of infection?

- What is your complication rate?

- Have you had any infections?

- How long have you been doing these procedures?

- Are you part of a clinical research registry collecting data on outcomes?

- Are you tracking and publishing your data in peer-reviewed medical journals?

The most qualified physicians publish their research findings in peer-reviewed journals. You can search their names on PubMed to see if they have published any of their results (*https://pubmed.ncbi.nlm.nih.gov/*) or are involved in any new intradiscal PRP studies (*https://clinicaltrials.gov/*). These studies may not only show their good results but also any complications they have had. Many physicians are reluctant to report their complications, but how will other physicians learn to avoid them if this information is not shared with the medical community at-large? Be diligent in your research and even ask to talk to a few patients of theirs that have had similar procedures to obtain insight as to their experience.

If you cannot find a reputable regenerative spine specialist in your area, you can also contact us at the Regenerative SportsCare Institute (RSI) (*https://www.regensportscare.com/*) where our team of regenerative spine specialists would look forward to evaluating your potential candidacy for intradiscal LR-PRP. We may also potentially know a reputable colleague of ours in your area.

It's taken over a decade to come up with our specific LR-PRP preparation, and our practice is the only center in the United States that currently has access to the use of the curved intradiscal delivery device. We have our own quality-control system to measure the cell counts of every patient we inject with PRP.

RSI is continually trying to improve our clinical outcomes through ongoing research, collaboration, and innovation. Few if any places in the world have as much experience as we have with this particular procedure. If you are far from the New York City area you may want to consider a telehealth visit with one of our regenerative spine specialists to judge your potential candidacy for intradiscal LR-PRP.

THE BENEFITS OF TELEHEALTH

Many people with chronic lower back pain searching for alternatives have tried conservative treatments and already have had their MRIs. These patients are in an ideal position to seek out second opinions via telehealth.

We've fully embraced telehealth at RSI. It's a great way for patients to get an opinion on whether or not to travel to New York City for intradiscal LR-PRP. Your MRI can be uploaded into our system, and one of our regen-erative spine specialists can review your history and imaging to see whether or not you are a good potential candidate before making the trip.

If you are deemed a good potential candidate, you would then travel to RSI and meet one of our physicians to perform a detailed physical examination and answer any remaining questions you might have regarding intradiscal LR-PRP. It's extremely important that you, the patient, feel completely comfortable with the spine specialist performing your procedure and that all of your questions are answered adequately prior to proceeding.

The final step is to then receive the intradiscal LR-PRP procedure. All of this could be accomplished in as little as a two-day visit to NYC.

Unfortunately, "Stem Cell" clinics have popped up all over the country, making unsubstantiated claims, thereby creating consumer confusion. Be very leery of any online ads luring you to remote clinics talking about amniotic products or cells from a source other than your own body. There is currently no sound scientific data that I know of to support any of their spurious claims. In addition, these types of treatments would not be FDA compliant unless they have successfully achieved regulatory clearance and have obtained an FDA claim to treat degenerative disc disease.

There are a multitude of cell products that are currently being injected into discs by physicians in the hopes of relieving CLBP, but the risks and benefits can differ vastly based on what is actually injected. To date, there are no FDA approved intradiscal regenerative treatments for patients with CLBP. This is one of the reasons that most insurance payers will not reimburse patients for these procedures—they deem them "experimental." It's also even more reason that you need to be as educated as you can be as a patient.

Patients that are searching for regenerative treatment options first need to understand the differences between autologous and allogeneic. The FDA regulates the use of these products:

- *Autologous products* are your own cells; they come from you, and they are processed on the same day, at the same facility, and put back into your body with what is referred to as "minimal manipulation." Physicians are not allowed to manipulate the cells with drugs or by culturing them in the lab. Physicians are also not allowed to transfer your cells to another individual. Your cells have to be used in your body for what is referred to as "homologous" use (i.e. for a similar purpose).

- *Allogeneic products* are cells from a source other than your own body, such as placental tissue or umbilical cord products. There is a great deal of controversy over these products, and the FDA does not currently allow them to be used in the United States unless they are used in an FDA approved clinical trial. Patients are being lured outside the US to try these treatments to get around the FDA regulatory issue. While there have been many companies conducting clinical trials to develop proprietary allogeneic cell products, no company has yet to show the FDA enough data to get approval to treat patients with CLBP in the US.

There are other concerns that you need to be made aware of with any allogeneic product. When you use cells other than your own, there's always a small risk for disease transmission or an immune reaction. In the United States, all allogeneic products go through a comprehensive screening process for transmissible diseases like hepatitis, AIDs, and other infectious conditions. But what most people are unaware of is a disease called **Creutzfeldt-Jakob disease or CJD**. CJD is also known as prion disease. It is a rare neurodegenerative disease that is invariably fatal. There is currently no way of screening for this, so therein lies the major risk with using any allogeneic cell products.

> *To the best of my knowledge, there is currently no scientific evidence of any intradiscal allogeneic product that shows superiority over the safer autologous LR-PRP you have learned about in this book.*

Therefore, it is my opinion that you should not take on the additional risk of these allogeneic products. What's more, many allogeneic products are often made not from a single donor but from pooled human tissue or blood products, meaning the risk for disease transmission from pooled tissue goes up significantly.

In the United States you are not allowed to use these allogeneic products unless you're doing a full FDA trial. The FDA and FTC are cracking down on companies trying to make treatment claims without going through the necessary regulatory processes.

It's important to keep this on your radar and understand the distinction between autologous and allogeneic products. Go to the most reputable regenerative spine specialist in your area, use your own cells first and keep it autologous. So now that you've decided to keep it autologous, you need to know that not all autologous products are the same.

The beauty of using your own stuff is that there is no risk for disease transmission, and it's personalized medicine at its best. Your DNA sequence is your own personalized code that you have lived with your whole life. That includes the composition of your platelets. You have your own unique blend of healing proteins that was especially designed to heal your tissue.

There's nothing safer than using your own cells, period.

Your capacity to heal is so much greater than you could ever imagine. Think about when you cut your skin—does it heal? Do you have to do anything for the healing to occur? It's completely on autopilot. Your cells are "naturally intelligent," and you were perfectly designed to heal yourself. When you heal your disc, your back pain will subside and you will be able to return to life.

Even if your physician is using autologous cells, there are still many different types that are currently being injected by clinicians into the disc, such as bone marrow aspirate, bone marrow concentrate, leukocyte-poor PRP, leukocyte-rich PRP, platelet lysate, adipose tissue, etc. Based on our experience and research, we believe the infection risk is the least with LR-PRP, and it is the only biologic that has DB RCT support and long-term outcomes data. We've used bone marrow concentrate in the past but noticed a slightly higher infection rate for reasons we do not yet fully understand.[50] There is also currently no scientific data to support the use of bone marrow concentrate over LR-PRP. So again, why take the additional risk?

We believe intradiscal LR-PRP is the safest intradiscal biologic with the most supportive preclinical and clinical data currently. This is based on our research and that of others, as well as twelve years of clinical experience performing these intradiscal procedures in well over one thousand patients.

At RSI we use only FDA 510k-cleared PRP kits and devices that we actually helped to invent to improve your safety and chances for success with these promising intradiscal procedures. While FDA cleared, these products are currently being used as what is referred to as "off label." The FDA does not regulate the practice of medicine. As a physician, in the confines of my practice I can use FDA-cleared devices in this off-label fashion, as long as I inform my patients of the potential risks and receive their informed consent.

To sum it up: search for a regenerative spine specialist using intradiscal LR-PRP who quantify their LR-PRP preparation with cell counts and are critically analyzing their outcomes with ongoing research.

WHAT TO EXPECT AT YOUR FIRST APPOINTMENT

Your physician should first listen to your symptoms and then ask direct questions: How did the pain start? What makes it better? What makes it worse? What tests have you had? Did another physician make a diagnosis already? Did they perform tests? How recent are those tests? Have the symptoms changed since those tests were done? What treatments have you had already? How did you respond to those treatments? How has CLBP changed your life? What activities would you look forward to returning to?

You want a physician who will actively listen to you without interrupting or staring off into a computer screen. Even if I think I know the answer based on the patient's intake questionnaire and a prior MRI, I still make sure I first listen intently. If you listen to your patients, they will tell you what's wrong with them. You don't want to be biased by another physician's assessment or the MRI report.

After your history has been obtained, your physician should perform a thorough physical exam of not only your spine, but also all of the surrounding joints, muscles, and nerves to make sure the pain is not coming from an arthritic hip or some other area outside of the spine that can mimic CLBP. A detailed neurologic exam will also be performed to look for weakness, numbness, or abnormal reflexes in your legs.

Finally, they should ask if you have any other concerns that you may not have expressed. This is very important in my experience; it's a question that helps me get to know my patients. Many patients have extreme anxiety over their current situation, and hopefully your physician can put things into perspective for you to allay some of these concerns. Clinical excellence—with compassion—is the trait you need to seek in your healthcare provider.

If you don't already have recent imaging of the spine (within six months), the next step would be to get an up-to-date MRI to see where your spine is in its current state. Like I previously mentioned, we often skip X-rays because of the radiation involved and go straight to the MRI as it offers so much more information. An MRI shows not only the bones that you see on an X-ray, but also the muscles, ligaments, nerves, discs, spinal canal, and joints—without any harmful radiation. While it's more costly, it's safer than other diagnostic tests and a necessary step towards being properly evaluated for intradiscal LR-PRP.

In certain circumstances, X-rays are still needed because most MRIs are performed while you're lying down so the spine is in an unloaded position. Performing standing X-rays will load the spine and may provide additional clues to hone in on your diagnosis. Standing X-rays with bending views are used to rule out spinal instability (abnormal shifting of the spinal segments on each other) which may require surgical stabilization.

WHO'S THE IDEAL CANDIDATE
FOR INTRADISCAL PRP?

Now that we have performed intradiscal LR-PRP injections for over a decade, we have learned a great deal...

The ideal candidate is someone who has moderate to severe lower back pain that's proven to be the result of degenerative disc disease that's lasted for more than three months and has been unresponsive to conservative treatments. The patient's MRI shows mild to moderate degeneration, not severe: no large disc herniation, no severe spinal stenosis, no severe scoliosis or severe slippage of the spine. Most patients have had an epidural steroid injection that gave them good but temporary relief.

In this scenario, most patients responded well to only one injection of LR-PRP, but if the relief is partial, I would consider a booster after six months. Almost every time we have repeated it, the patient has had further improvement. We have not had to repeat the procedure more than twice in any one patient to achieve long-term improvement.

WHAT TO EXPECT WITH AN
INTRADISCAL LR-PRP PROCEDURE

The majority of these procedures can be performed safely as an outpatient. The procedure is usually only sixty minutes long, but you are at the facility for about two-to-three hours between setup and recovery. Here are the typical patient steps at RSI:

The patient arrives and gets prepared for the procedure. An intravenous line is started so that we can administer light sedation during the procedure. Not every intradiscal PRP procedure has to be performed with sedation, but the majority of patients prefer it this way in our experience.

The patient is then brought to the procedure suite where we draw their blood under sterile conditions right before the procedure. The blood is placed in our FDA approved kits. A small amount of baseline blood and a small amount of PRP are then sent to the lab for cell count testing for quality control and dosing.

While the blood is spinning in the centrifuge (approximately fifteen minutes), we prepare you for the procedure by placing you comfortably on your stomach on the procedure table.

Using fluoroscopy, we mark out the spinal levels we are going to be treating. You are then sedated.

We then begin to clean the skin, drape the area of interest, and apply local anesthetic. Even though you are sedated, the local anesthesia is still helpful to make the insertion of the needles painless.

Intradiscal curved catheters are then guided precisely into the discs that need treatment under fluoroscopic guidance. By this time, the LR-PRP is ready for injection. We are the only facility in the US that has access to the curved catheter technique. We believe using the curved catheter to precisely deliver the LR-PRP offers potential advantages over the typical straight-needle technique used by other centers; however, further research is needed to study its effects.

We first inject a small amount of contrast agent to make sure we are filling the tears in the disc. We also inject a minute amount of antibiotics to prevent infection. We've learned that injecting a small amount of a safe anesthetic into the disc significantly reduces post-procedure pain. We are careful to keep these amounts to a minimum so that the majority of the injection is the LR-PRP. The disc can only hold maybe a total of three teaspoons of additional volume.

Then over the course of a few minutes, we gently fill each degenerated disc with the LR-PRP. Usually this amounts to about two teaspoons of the LR-PRP per disc.

The needles and catheters are then removed, and a small bandage is placed on the injection sites. The patient is then brought to the recovery room and monitored for sixty minutes for any adverse reactions.

Then the patient is discharged home with instructions. We advise taking 48–72 hours off from work. Oral pain medication is prescribed only for the first few days.

This procedure is extremely safe and efficient when performed by competent physicians. It does not need to be performed in a hospital, but it does need to be performed in a clean and safe fluoroscopy procedure suite. While sedation is not an absolute, it provides the patient with a more comfortable procedure experience as injecting into degenerative discs can be painful. The pressure of injecting into painful tears in the disc can temporarily trigger your typical back spasms. These spasms will usually subside in three days.

In the state of New York, a facility needs added qualification to offer anesthesia in the outpatient setting by a board-certified anesthesiologist. At RSI, we have obtained and maintained this additional accreditation through the American Association for Accreditation of Ambulatory Surgery Facilities. While this took a great deal of time and effort, it was important for us to be able to offer our patients safe, high-quality care in the more cost-effective outpatient clinical setting.

Hopefully, the information in this chapter has given you a framework to make an educated decision for yourself or a loved one suffering from CLBP. If you have any further questions, you could always contact us at RSI.

In the final chapter of this book, I will sum it all up and provide you with a glimpse of where I believe we are going with spinecare.

CHAPTER 10

THE FUTURE OF SPINECARE

"The most reliable way to predict the future is to create it."

—**ABRAHAM LINCOLN**, 1809–1865

Lower back pain should be nothing more than a hiccup in life, not the wrecking ball it has been for so many. Unfortunately, our traditional treatments of drugs and surgery have failed to "fix" the lower back pain problem. Patients are beginning to recognize the advantages, the safety, the efficiency, and the increasing effectiveness that regenerative medicine offers. Regenerative spinecare is coming for the simple reason it is the right thing for patients.

Our healthcare system has historically

*overcomplicated the CLBP problem and
mismanaged patients for decades.*

It has placed patients at unnecessary risk with poorly conceived, ineffectual treatments that have wasted precious healthcare resources. Drugs and surgery typically are only palliative treatments because they do not address the root causes of why discs degenerate. While some patients experience temporary improvement, frequently the back pain returns and worsens over time. This is why CLBP is a pandemic in its own right and our inability to solve this problem has only contributed to the opioid epidemic in the United States.

We need to shift our thinking toward viewing the disc as the "heart" of the spine. The spine community needs to move away from treating CLBP patients with rods, plates, screws, and narcotics and toward treatments that heal and preserve the disc. I strongly believe if we shift the treatment paradigm toward regenerative medicine, we will have a chance to preserve the spine and end back pain for many. Regenerative medicine will help us gracefully transition out of the "management" stage of degenerative disc disease and into the "cure" stage.

It has been illuminating to finally identify new and potentially reversible factors contributing to degenerative disc disease that we can target with nothing more than a concentration of your own healing cells and proteins. However, you must be your own advocate and perform your own research. Remember, *effective treatment begins with an accurate diagnosis.* It's important that you seek out the right medical provider from the beginning, one who will spend time listening to your history, performing a thorough physical exam, reviewing your images with you so you understand your condition, and who will start with the least invasive treatments before considering any surgery. Which practitioner you see at the beginning of your treatment path can really make a difference in your final outcome.

Suffering for years with CLBP can be terrifying and life altering. Many patients that I see are scared and feel "broken." *Chronic lower back pain is nothing more than an unhealed wound— so let's just heal it.* Your body has an amazing capacity to heal itself with minimal intervention.

> The simple fact I hope to convey in this book is:
> everything you need to get better is already inside you.

You are essentially your own "drug store." As a regenerative spine specialist, we need to concentrate your healing cells and proteins and place them precisely where the root of the problem is to get you back to life. Sometimes the solutions to such complex problems can be so elegant and simple—this is one of those instances. We are entering an exciting new era in personalized medicine, the "Age of Biology," where previously incurable conditions like degenerative disc disease may be cured with regenerative medicine.

We are only now beginning to better understand the micro-environment of the disc, its inability to heal on its own, and the potential role that bacteria play in degenerative disc disease. There are differences in different PRP preparations that matter—*remember: the spine has a microbiome.* It wasn't until recently that studies demonstrated the role that the balance of bacteria play, not only in our general health, but also in the health of our spines. It is now believed that the discs, like our guts, have their own intradiscal microbiome, with many different bacteria present even in a normal disc. It is believed that the overgrowth of certain types of bacteria (dysbiosis) may be contributing to degenerative disc disease.

That may be why intradiscal LR-PRP has been so safe and successful in our practice at RSI. It is possible that LR-PRP may be doing more than just healing painful tears in the disc wall. We may actually be killing two birds with one stone. These LR-PRP cell preparations also contain a high concentration of our bacteria-fighting white blood cells, which have been shown to suppress the overgrowth of certain bacteria now believed to actually cause degenerative disc disease—*C. Acnes.* Yes, this is the same organism that is responsible for acne. I often told my patients in the past that your disc protrusion is analogous to a painful pimple, not fully understanding the truth behind those words.

Regenerative medicine can save your spine, but unfortunately this field of medicine has been largely unregulated, and navigating it requires a bit of caveat emptor—"buyer beware." Stem cell clinics are popping up all over the country, making exaggerated or false claims. Patients cannot be naive when it comes to their healthcare and must take special care when it comes to this emerging field of regenerative medicine. Hence one of my major motivations to write this book is to share my knowledge to help you become better informed as you navigate through these regenerative treatment options. Do your homework to find the best regenerative spine specialist in your area. It's my hope that after reading this book you are prepared to be your own advocate and use the resources provided to make more informed healthcare decisions.

The global clinical unmet need is significant and, as of the writing of this book, LR-PRP is, in my opinion, our current best solution to the CLBP problem. Its simplicity makes it well-suited to scale to meet this large and growing global clinical need. While I have seen many new and promising back pain treatments come and go, this treatment has staying power because it is a root-cause treatment for degenerative disc disease. It's so important for you or a loved one suffering from CLBP to become aware of this treatment option that is readily available today with the right provider.

Putting together the material for this book has given me a chance to reflect on not only those patient experiences that have shaped me, but also those experiences outside of medicine that have enlightened me. Who would have thought that having a farm and being exposed to some creative and innovative farmers and veterinarians would lead me to a potential cure and strategy to create a treatment paradigm shift in how we manage CLBP?

While many companies are searching for proprietary cell preparations or pharmaceuticals to treat degenerative disc disease, it will be difficult in my opinion to mimic what the body has evolved to do so well on its own over thousands of years.

The shift towards using regenerative medicine solutions for CLBP is already underway, and it is so important that we all collaborate to make these treatments as simple, safe, and effective as we can. Our approach is to harness your body's innate ability to heal by injecting billions of your platelets and millions of your white blood cells directly into painful non-healing tears inside your disc. In this time of evolving personalized and precision medicine, what could be more personalized and precise than the use of your own cells to heal your disc? Talk about democratizing a treatment for all —there is nothing proprietary about using your own stuff!

> *Like my dad told me, "Keep focused on where you want to go. Don't feel that you need to quiet all of the barking dogs along the way."*

There are many barriers to new treatments in medicine. There are scientific, regulatory, financial, reimbursement, and political barriers. It will take a great deal of momentum to disrupt entrenched players that rely too heavily on income from spinal fusion surgery. This shift will only occur through a healthcare system that is built on a foundation of vertical collaboration that puts the needs of the patient first. The time is right for this shift to occur. I believe that regenerative medicine has the ability to gracefully transition our healthcare system from the "management" stage to the "cure" stage of treatment for degenerative disc disease.

Our historic treatments focused on "symptom-modifying therapies," while what we needed all along were "structure-modifying therapies" like intradiscal LR-PRP.

Not only does regenerative medicine offer better patient care, it offers significant value to healthcare systems. Imagine the potential savings created by regenerative treatments that are a fraction of the cost of spinal surgery with significantly less risk and recovery time. Most patients we treat return to work in only a few days. Since spinal implants are not used in regenerative procedures, the infection risk is that much lower, while also offering an opioid-sparing treatment option.

> *Our healthcare system is in desperate need of a creative solution to the back pain pandemic—like intradiscal LR-PRP.*

This is the future of spinecare: value based, minimally invasive, opioid-sparing, regenerative treatments that halt or reverse degenerative disc, scaled through specialized outpatient clinics like RSI. We have both a social and an ethical prerogative to create a sustainable solution for patients with CLBP. There is a need, now more than ever, for patients to reconnect on a personal level with their healthcare providers. It's easier to create these vertical cooperatives at the small specialty clinic level because it is about building personal relationships. Too big is often too impersonal in my opinion.

As exciting as it has been to discover potentially new and reversible factors that we can target with our regenerative treatments, our work is not done. These treatments have room for improvement and optimization. We have collaborated with industry partners to invent a new and optimized PRP delivery system that we believe is ideal for the treatment of degenerative disc disease. It combines a new delivery device and PRP kit that is able to achieve significantly higher concentration of platelets delivered precisely to the annulus fibrosus. Higher concentration LR-PRP coupled with more precise delivery I believe will further improve our clinical outcomes. Now that these new devices have achieved 510(k) clearance from the FDA, we are able to begin the next round of clinical studies.

This optimized system is the culmination of over a decade of clinical experience and research. That is the way new discoveries in medicine advance, through vertical collaboration and innovation. We are very excited to see how this translates into better outcomes for patients with degenerative disc disease.

As there is little if any industry support for autologous cell therapies, we have created the Regenerative SportsCare

Foundation (RSF), a 501(c)(3) charitable organization whose mission is to cure degenerative disc disease. If you would like to keep abreast of our research, please go to: (https://www .regensportscare.com/foundation/).

Seek out a regenerative spine specialist who is well-versed in intradiscal LR-PRP. Please know that many physicians and researchers around the globe are well aware of the short-comings of our current treatments for CLBP. These professionals are stretching our thinking and vision to create a transformational change for the better in how we manage this vexatious healthcare problem so that it does not have to become chronic for you.

It is my sincere hope that this book has given you the information you need to make an informed choice on how to better manage your CLBP, and "choice" is the key word here. Remember, you always have a choice when it comes to your personal healthcare. If you or a loved one is frustrated with the care you are receiving, let the information you've learned from this book guide you forward into a new and more positive direction. Intradiscal LR-PRP offers many patients suffering from CLBP a simple and safe new approach to help *Heal Your Disc & End Your Pain.*

DISCLAIMER

The U.S. Food & Drug Administration (FDA) does not regulate the practice of medicine. However, it does have regulatory and oversight responsibility for products used in regenerative medicine therapy such as Regenerative SportsCare Institute's (RSI) Autologous Cell Therapy and Plasma Rich Protein Therapy. Given the nature of the substances used in RSI's therapies (patients' own blood and cells) and/or how the substances are handled by RSI during the procedures, the FDA does not require RSI to obtain premarket review and approval for these procedures. Thus, RSI's procedures are not FDA approved, and you will need to determine whether the particular RSI procedure you are considering is right for you in consultation with your own medical professional.

The devices used by RSI during the procedures are FDA 510 (k) cleared for use in indications and procedures different from that of RSI. As permitted by the FDA, RSI and its physicians are using these FDA-cleared devices for RSI procedures in an off-label manner, according to their best knowledge and judgment, based on sound medical evidence, and in the best interest of their patients.

As with any medical treatment, no guarantees or claim of cures are made as to the extent of the response to treatment. Results vary from patient to patient, even with a similar diagnosis, as the body's internal status is unique to each individual patient. Patient results and stories in this book, while real, may not be typical. Because of this fact, RSI cannot offer, infer, or suggest that there is any certainty of any given outcome in your treatment.

ACKNOWLEDGMENTS

First I would like to acknowledge my wonderful team who left the comfort and security of a major hospital and took a chance to join me in creating this new platform of musculoskeletal healthcare at RSI. Without their dedication to patient care, the medical discoveries you have read about in this book would never have been possible. Maria Duran, our practice manager, is a gentle and kind leader. Pamela Harrelson, our office manager, is loyal to the core and always has the patient's best interest at heart. Beatriz Jimenez, our patient care coordinator, like her mother, Maria, is gentle and kind, but she also brings a sense of calming humor to the office. Allen Chambers, our Director of Radiology, has been with me for most of my career, assisting me in all of our interventional procedures seamlessly. Michael Ferrari, our MRI/radiology technician, calmly guides our patients through their procedures with encouragement and compassion. Chris Contingjo and Naomi Kho, our nurses, adeptly handle all aspects of patient care, and Anthony Harrelson, who keeps

RSI spotless. It's my honor to work with all of you and appreciate all your efforts to treat our patients with respect and dignity.

Then there are my colleagues at RSI who've also left the mothership to explore this emerging field of regenerative orthopedic medicine together. Dr. Christopher Lutz, my brother, has practiced side by side with me now for over two decades, taking care of our patients, teaching our fellows, performing research, and discussing innovative ways of doing things better. As you have read, we come from a family with medical roots that run deep. Chris is also an exemplary physician with a big heart who also has the highest integrity and competency. One of my colleagues from HSS, Dr. Jennifer Solomon, joined us in the middle of the pandemic. Jennifer is a patient advocate extraordinaire and a gifted energetic physician. More recently, another one of my colleagues from HSS has joined RSI, Dr. Elizabeth Manejias, our functional medicine expert. The combination of regenerative medicine and functional medicine is extremely powerful and is going to change healthcare for the better. Having caring and competent colleagues all working together to put the needs of our patients first makes RSI a very special place.

To Dr. Avishai Neuman, the medical director of Centurion

Anesthesia, thanks for all you and your fine group of anesthesiologists do to help our intradiscal PRP patients have a safe and comfortable experience with their procedures.

A special thank you to Kevin Towers, DPT, for helping our intradiscal PRP patients rehabilitate not just back to their previous levels of activities but beyond. Kevin takes a very scientific approach to exercise that our patients have benefitted from greatly. There is an art to gradually loading healing discs that Kevin has mastered.

I would like to acknowledge all of our intradiscal orthobiologic patients who ventured into uncharted waters with me. Medical discoveries have to start somewhere, and they usually begin with a trusting doctor-patient relationship. Without your willingness to try these relatively unproven treatments, we never would have obtained the knowledge of their tremendous benefit. I am in awe of your courage and humbled to be your physician.

To all my colleagues at HSS, I have a tremendous amount of respect for you and your dedication to patient care, teaching, and research. HSS is a very special place and will always hold a warm spot in my heart. A special acknowledgment to Dr. Russell F. Warren, Surgeon-in-Chief emeritus at HSS, thank you for the opportunity to establish the Physiatry Department. Without your support and guidance, I am not sure it would have happened. You are a one-of-a-kind visionary leader. I would also like to acknowledge Dr. Joseph Feinberg and Dr. Joel Press for their leadership in taking the HSS Physiatry Department to the next level.

I would like to acknowledge the many teachers and professors over the years that have contributed to my growth. The road to becoming a physician is a long one. Teaching is such a noble profession that is so often underappreciated. A very special thank you to my high school science teacher, Mike Generallo, for literally "planting the seed" of biology in my mind. Teaching me how to connect the scientific dots has led me to the discovery of intradiscal **LR-PRP** as a root cause treatment for degenerative disc disease.

I would like to acknowledge my team at Orthobond Corporation, especially Dr. Meredith Prysak and Dr. Jordan Katz. They have educated me on the role that bacteria play not only with regards to medical device failure but also in degenerative disc disease. We have a brilliant team of scientists and business executives dedicated to improving the safety of medical devices by reducing the risk of biofilm formation through a novel antimicrobial nanosurface.

I want to acknowledge the family foundations that have provided financial support to our research in regenerative medicine: Thomas Kempner, Eileen Farbman, Michael Vranos, and Stephen Schwarzman. Without their generous contributions, we would not have been able to create the Regenerative SportsCare Foundation (RSF) and continue our research. Our research team consists of many different individuals that are all collaborating to advance the field of regenerative medicine: Dr. Meredith Prysak, Dr. Jennifer Cheng, Dr. Daniel Kuebler, Tylor Zukovsky, Cole Lutz, Dr. Mairin Jerome, Dr. Christopher Kyriakides, and Mohammed Sharaf.

To my innovation team, Andy McGillicuddy, Barry Zimble, Cameron Keefe, and Annette Fagnant, it's such a pleasure working with individuals who are creative, competent, and not just concerned about making profits. I'm looking forward to seeing the impact our inventions will have on improving patient care.

To my colleague Dr. Chris Centeno, the Chief Medical Officer of Regenexx, I have a tremendous amount of respect for your efforts in establishing interventional orthopedics and regenerative medicine as a new platform of musculo-skeletal care.

When I decided to write a book, I didn't know where to start. If it weren't for Tracey Merz, my son Cole's fiancée, I don't think this book would have gotten off the ground. Tracey is Mel Robbins's Senior Content Manager and provided me with invaluable insights into how to organize and launch this book.

Tracey also led me to my amazing team at Scribe: Mikey Kershisnik, my lead publishing manager, whose energy and follow-through has kept me on point; Janet Murnaghan, my scribe, who interviewed me and helped me compose my thoughts in an organized fashion; Kelly Teemer, my senior strategy specialist; and Teresa Muniz, my cover designer.

To my friends Peter Scaturro, Lisa D'Urso, Khalil Barrage, and David Helfet, it's easy to take the road less traveled when you have such supportive friends who've got your back. Your friendship, business acumen, and guidance mean a great deal to me. Peter is taking a more active business role to help RSI become a model platform for musculoskeletal care. I'm so glad you are involved in helping us move this platform of care forward so more patients can benefit.

I would now like to acknowledge my special family. It started with my parents, Elmar and Barbara, who met in the emergency room at St. Mary's hospital in Passaic, New Jersey, in the late 1950s. Dad was a physician, and Mom was a nurse. Not only did they love us with all their hearts, but they educated us by their example of what a gift it is to become a healer. All four of us became physicians. My sister Mary Bernadette is a pediatrician in New Jersey, and my other brother Michael is a dermatologic surgeon in Florida. Without our parents' example, we all wouldn't be the physicians we are today.

Then there are my own children, Cole, Olivia, Anna, and my son-in-law Paul. It's an amazing thing when your adult children show a genuine interest in what you are doing. Each one of them not only encouraged me to write this book, but they also read the draft and contributed to its content. They corrected my many grammatical errors (they are well-educated Laurentians), and also told it straight when things just didn't make sense. I love you all and am so proud of the young adults you have become.

Finally, to my wife, Paula, what can I say? You have been an unending source of love and support right from the start of our relationship, and it just keeps growing. Your beauty, integrity, and intelligence inspire me. It was Paula, a certified functional medicine health coach, who first brought to my attention the role that the microbiome plays in overall health and disease. I would also like to share some of the pivotal acts of love she has performed to support my professional growth over the years.

In medical school, when I was applying for my residency, I was initially rejected by the Mayo Clinic. It was Paula who, unbeknownst to me, wrote a letter on my behalf expressing my continued interest in their program. It eventually worked out because of her, despite my obstinance. When I was disillusioned about physiatry and was reconsidering orthopedic surgery, she urged me to stick with it and see it through. When I was offered the position at HSS to start a Physiatry Department, knowing quite well that more home responsibilities would fall on her, she said to go for it. When I wanted to create RSI, we both had to sign a substantial bank loan to make it happen. Paula filled in wherever necessary to bring RSI where it is today. Finally, when I recently got caught in a riptide at Miami Beach and almost drowned, it was Paula who alerted the lifeguards to save me. My success is your success. I love you with all of my heart, and it is a privilege to be enjoying this journey with you!

ABOUT THE AUTHOR

DR. GREGORY LUTZ is the Founder of the Regenerative SportsCare Institute, Physiatrist-in-Chief Emeritus at Hospital for Special Surgery, and a professor of clinical rehabilitation medicine at Weill Medical College of Cornell University. A pioneer in regenerative orthopedic medicine, Dr. Lutz has co-authored more than sixty scientific publications, including the first double-blind, randomized, controlled study demonstrating the clinical efficacy of intradiscal platelet-rich plasma therapy. Dr. Lutz is a former board member of the Interventional OrthoBiologics Foundation and the Co-Founder and Executive Chairman of Orthobond Corporation.

ENDNOTES

1   Mark B. Kabins and James N. Weinstein, "The History of Vertebral Screw and Pedicle Screw Fixation," *The Iowa Orthopaedic Journal* 11 (1991): 127–136, https://www.ncbi.nlm.nih.gov/pmc/articles/PMC 2328959/.

2   GBD 2017 Disease and Injury Incidence and Prevalence Collaborators, "Global, Regional, and National Incidence, Prevalence, and Years Lived with Disability for 354 Diseases and Injuries for 195 Countries and Territories, 1990–2017: A Systematic Analysis for the Global Burden of Disease Study 2017," *Lancet* 392, no. 10159 (November 2018): 1789–1858, https://doi.org/10.1016/S0140-6736(18)32279-7.

3   Richard A. Deyo, Michael Von Korff, and David Duhrkoop, "Opioids for Low Back Pain," *The BMJ* 2015, no. 350 (January 5, 2015): g6380, https://doi.org/10.1136/bmj.g6380.

4   "Opioid Data Analysis and Resources," US Centers for Disease Control and Prevention, last modified June 1, 2022, https://www.cdc.gov/opioids /data/analysis-resources.html.

5   US Centers for Disease Control and Prevention, *2018 Annual Surveillance Report of Drug-Related Risks and Outcomes* (Atlanta: CDC, US Department of Health and Human Services, August 31, 2018), 51, https://www.cdc .gov/drugoverdose/pdf/pubs/2018-cdc-drug-surveillance-report.pdf.

6   Yu Tung Lo et al., "Long-Term Opioid Prescriptions after Spine Surgery: A Meta-Analysis of Prevalence and Risk Factors," *World Neurosurgery* 141 (September 2020): e894–e920, https://doi.org/10.1016/j.wneu.2020.06 .081.

7   Hansen Deng et al., "Elective Lumbar Fusion in the United States: National Trends in Inpatient Complications and Cost from 2002–2014," *Journal of Neurosurgical Sciences* 65, no. 5 (October 2021): 503–512, https://doi.org/10.23736/S0390-5616.19.04647-2.

8   Trang H. Nguyen et al., "Long-Term Outcomes of Lumbar Fusion among Workers' Compensation Subjects: A Historical Cohort Study," *Spine* 36, no. 4 (February 15, 2011): 320–331, https://doi.org/10.1097/BRS.0b013e3181ccc220.

9   Institute of Medicine Committee on Advancing Pain Research, Care, and Education, *Relieving Pain in America: A Blueprint for Transforming Prevention, Care, Education, and Research* (Washington, DC: National Academies Press, 2011), 5, https://doi.org/10.17226/13172.

10 Matthias Pumberger et al., "Perioperative Mortality after Lumbar Spinal Fusion Surgery: An Analysis of Epidemiology and Risk Factors," *European Spine Journal* 21, no. 8 (August 2012): 1633–1639, https://doi.org/10.1007/s00586-012-2298-8.

11 Joseph L. Dieleman et al., "US Health Care Spending by Payer and Health Condition, 1996–2016," *JAMA* 323, no. 9 (March 3, 2020): 863–884, https://doi.org/10.1001/jama.2020.0734.

12 Amir Qaseem et al., "Noninvasive Treatments for Acute, Subacute, and Chronic Low Back Pain: A Clinical Practice Guideline from the American College of Physicians," *Annals of Internal Medicine* 166, no. 7 (April 4, 2017): 514–530, https://doi.org/10.7326/M16-2367.

13 Matthew Smuck et al., "Smoking Is Associated with Pain in All Body Regions, with Greatest Influence on Spinal Pain," *Pain Medicine* 21, no. 9 (September 2020): 1759–1768, https://doi.org/10.1093/pm/pnz224.

14 Serge Renaud et al., "Platelet Function after Cigarette Smoking in Relation to Nicotine and Carbon Monoxide," *Clinical Pharmacology and Therapeutics* 36, no. 3 (September 1984): 389–395, https://doi.org/10.1038/clpt.1984.193.

15 Ronald Donelson, Greg McIntosh, and Hamilton Hall, "Is It Time to Rethink the Typical Course of Low Back Pain?," *Physical Medicine and*

Rehabilitation 4, no. 6 (June 2012): 394–401, https://doi.org/10.1016/j.pmrj.2011.10.015.

16 KenYong-Hing and William H. Kirkaldy-Willis, "The Pathophysiology of Degenerative Disease of the Lumbar Spine," *Orthopedic Clinics of North America* 14, no. 3 (July 1983): 491–504, https://doi.org/10.1016/S0030-5898(20)31329-8.

17 Zhi Y. Kho and Sunil K. Lal, "The Human Gut Microbiome—A Potential Controller of Wellness and Disease," *Frontiers in Microbiology* 9 (August 14, 2018): 1835, https://doi.org/10.3389/fmicb.2018.01835.

18 Hanne B. Albert et al., "Antibiotic Treatment in Patients with Chronic Low Back Pain and Vertebral Bone Edema (Modic Type 1 Changes): A Double-Blind Randomized Clinical Controlled Trial of Efficacy," *European Spine Journal* 22, no. 4 (April 2013): 697–707, https://doi.org/10.1007/s00586-013-2675-y.

19 Zhe Chen et al., "Modic Changes and Disc Degeneration Caused by Inoculation of *Propionibacterium acnes* inside Intervertebral Discs of Rabbits: A Pilot Study," *BioMed Research International* 2016, no. 9612437 (January 26, 2016), https://doi.org/10.1155/2016/9612437.

20 Shanmuganathan Rajasekaran et al., "Human Intervertebral Discs Harbour a Unique Microbiome and Dysbiosis Determines Health and Disease," *European Spine Journal* 29, no. 7 (July 2020): 1621–1640, https://doi.org/10.1007/s00586-020-06446-z.

21 Hansen Deng et al., "Elective Lumbar Fusion in the United States: National Trends in Inpatient Complications and Cost from 2002–2014," *Journal of Neurosurgical Sciences* 65, no. 5 (October 2021): 503–512, https://doi.org/10.23736/S0390-5616.19.04647-2.

22 T. F. Moriarty, D. W. Grainger, and R. G. Richards, "Challenges in Linking Preclinical Anti-Microbial Research Strategies with Clinical Outcomes for Device-Associated Infections," *European Cells and Materials* 28 (September 12, 2014): 112–128, https://doi.org/10.22203/ecm.v028a09.

23 Anthony G. Gristina, Paul T. Naylor, and Quentin Myrvik, "Infections from Biomaterials and Implants: A Race for the Surface," *Medical*

Progress through Technology 14, no. 3-4 (1988): 205–224,
https://pubmed.ncbi.nlm.nih.gov/2978593/.

24 Suganthan Veerachamy et al., "Bacterial Adherence and Biofilm
Formation on Medical Implants: A Review," *Proceedings of the Institution
of Mechanical Engineers, Part H: Journal of Engineering in Medicine* 228,
no. 10 (October 2014): 1083–1099, https://doi.org/10.1177/0954411
914556137.

25 Michael E. Steinhaus et al., "Risk Factors for Positive Cultures in
Presumed Aseptic Revision Spine Surgery," *Spine* 44, no. 3 (February
2019): 177–184, https://doi.org/10.1097/BRS.0000000000002792.

26 Tucker C. Callanan et al., "Prevalence of Occult Infections in Posterior
Instrumented Spinal Fusion," *Clinical Spine Surgery* 34, no. 1 (February
2021): 25–31, https://doi.org/10.1097/BSD.0000000000001014.

27 Daniel Karczewski et al., "Implications for Diagnosis and Treatment
of Peri-Spinal Implant Infections from Experiences in Periprosthetic
Joint Infections—A Literature Comparison and Review,"
Journal of Spine Surgery 6, no. 4 (December 2020): 800–813,
https://doi.org/10.21037/jss-20-12.

28 Lukas Leitner et al., "Pedicle Screw Loosening Is Correlated to
Chronic Subclinical Deep Implant Infection: A Retrospective Database
Analysis," *European Spine Journal* 27, no. 10 (October 2018): 2529–2535,
https://doi.org/10.1007/s00586-018-5592-2; Matthias Pumberger et
al., "Unexpected Positive Cultures in Presumed Aseptic Revision Spine
Surgery Using Sonication," *The Bone and Joint Journal* 101-B, no. 5
(May 2019): 621–624, https://doi.org/10.1302/0301-620X.101B5
.BJJ-2018-1168.R1.

29 Vincent Prinz et al., "High Frequency of Low-Virulent Microorganisms
Detected by Sonication of Pedicle Screws: A Potential Cause for Implant
Failure," *Journal of Neurosurgery* 31, no. 3 (May 28, 2019): 424–429,
https://doi.org/10.3171/2019.1.SPINE181025.

30 Simon Thomson, "Failed Back Surgery Syndrome—Definition,
Epidemiology and Demographics," *British Journal of Pain* 7, no. 1
(February 2013): 56–59, https://doi.org/10.1177/2049463713479096.

[31]   Nicholas R. Beatty et al., "Spondylodiscitis Due to Cutibacterium acnes following Lumbosacral Intradiscal Biologic Therapy: A Case Report," *Regenerative Medicine* 14, no. 9 (September 2019): 823–829, https://doi.org/10.2217/rme-2019-0008.

[32]   Koji Akeda et al., "Platelet-Rich Plasma Stimulates Porcine Articular Chondrocyte Proliferation and Matrix Biosynthesis," *Osteoarthritis and Cartilage* 14, no. 12 (December 2006): 1272–1280, https://doi.org/10.1016/j.joca.2006.05.008.

[33]   Koji Akeda et al., "Platelet-Rich Plasma (PRP) Stimulates the Extracellular Matrix Metabolism of Porcine Nucleus Pulposus and Anulus Fibrosus Cells Cultured in Alginate Beads," *Spine* 31, no. 9 (April 20, 2006): 959–966, https://doi.org/10.1097/01.brs.0000214942.78119.24.

[34]   Wei-Hong Chen et al., "Tissue-Engineered Intervertebral Disc and Chondrogenesis Using Human Nucleus Pulposus Regulated through TGF-Beta1 in Platelet-Rich Plasma," *Journal of Cellular Physiology* 209, no. 3 (December 2006): 744–754, https://doi.org/10.1002/jcp.20765.

[35]   Yetsa A. Tuakli-Wosornu et al., "Lumbar Intradiskal Platelet-Rich Plasma (PRP) Injections: A Prospective, Double-Blind, Randomized Controlled Study," *Physical Medicine and Rehabilitation* 8, no. 1 (January 2016): 1–10, https://doi.org/10.1016/j.pmrj.2015.08.010.

[36]   Michael Monfett et al., "Intradiscal Platelet-Rich Plasma (PRP) Injections for Discogenic Low Back Pain: An Update," *International Orthopaedics* 40, no. 6 (June 2016): 1321–1328, https://doi.org/10.1007/s00264-016-3178-3; Jennifer Cheng et al., "Treatment of Symptomatic Degenerative Intervertebral Discs with Autologous Platelet-Rich Plasma: Follow-Up at 5–9 Years," *Regenerative Medicine* 14, no. 9 (September 2019): 831–840, https://doi.org/10.2217/rme-2019-0040.

[37]   Koji Akeda et al, 2019. "Platelet-Rich Plasma in the Management of Chronic Low Back Pain: A Critical Review." *Journal of Pain Research* 12, (2019), 753-767.

[38]   Koji Akeda et al, "Platelet-Rich Plasma-Releasate (PRPr) for the Treatment of Discogenic Low Back Pain Patients: Long-Term Follow-Up

Survey," *Medicina (Kaunas) 58*, (March 2022): 428. doi:10.3390/medicina58030428.

39 Koji Akeda et al, "Platelet-Rich Plasma Releasate versus Corticosteroid for the Treatment of Discogenic Low Back Pain: A Double-Blind Randomized Controlled Trial," J Clin Med, (January 2022): 304. doi:10.3390/jcm11020304.

40 M.O. Schepers et al, "Effectiveness of intradiscal platelet rich plasma for discogenic low back pain without Modic changes: A randomized controlled trial," Intervent Pain Med, (2022). doi.org/10.1016/j.inpm.2022.100011

41 Shuji Obata et al., "Effect of Autologous Platelet-Rich Plasma-Releasate on Intervertebral Disc Degeneration in the Rabbit Anular Puncture Model: A Preclinical Study," *Arthritis Research and Therapy* 14, no. 6 (November 5, 2012): R241, https://doi.org/10.1186/ar4084.

42 Meredith H. Prysak et al., "A Retrospective Analysis of a Commercially Available Platelet-Rich Plasma Kit during Clinical Use," *Physical Medicine and Rehabilitation* 13, no. 12 (December 2021): 1410–1417, https://doi.org/10.1002/pmrj.12569.

43 Cole Lutz et al., "Clinical Outcomes following Intradiscal Injections of Higher-Concentration Platelet-Rich Plasma in Patients with Chronic Lumbar Discogenic Pain," *International Orthopaedics* 46, no. 6 (June 2022): 1381–1385, https://doi.org/10.1007/s00264-022-05389-y.

44 Mairin A. Jerome, Christopher Lutz, and Gregory E. Lutz, "Risks of Intradiscal Orthobiologic Injections: A Review of the Literature and Case Series Presentation," *International Journal of Spine Surgery* 15, no. s1 (April 2021): 26–39, https://doi.org/10.14444/8053.

45 Meredith H. Prysak et al., "Optimizing the Safety of Intradiscal Platelet-Rich Plasma: An *In Vitro* Study with *Cutibacterium acnes*," *Regenerative Medicine* 14, no. 10 (October 2019): 955–967, https://doi.org/10.2217/rme-2019-0098.

46 Sylvia Hondke, "Proliferation, Migration, and ECM Formation Potential of Human Annulus Fibrosus Cells Is Independent of

Degeneration Status," *Cartilage* 11, no. 2, (April 2022): 192-202. doi:10.1177/1947603518764265.

[47] JR Warren and B Marshall, "Unidentified curved bacilli on gastric epithelium in active chronic gastritis," *Lancet 1*. (June 1983): 1273-5. PMID: 6134060.

[48] Aleksandra Sokic-Milutinovic et al, "Role of Helicobacter pylori infection in gastric carcinogenesis: Current knowledge and future directions," *World J Gastroenterol 11*, (November 2017): 11654-72. doi:10.3748/wjg.v21.i41.11654.

[49] Barry Marshall and Paul C. Adams, "*Helicobacter pylori*: A Nobel Pursuit?," *Canadian Journal of Gastroenterology and Hepatology* 22, no. 11 (November 2008): 895–896, https://doi.org/10.1155/2008/459810.

[50] Mairin A. Jerome, Christopher Lutz, and Gregory E. Lutz, "Risks of Intradiscal Orthobiologic Injections: A Review of the Literature and Case Series Presentation," *International Journal of Spine Surgery* 15, no. s1 (April 2021): 26–39, https://doi.org/10.14444/8053.

9 781544 537221